# Good Enough Mothering?

Lone mothers and their children currently comprise almost 20 per cent of all families with dependent children in Britain. Their numbers have nearly trebled since 1970. In Europe and in the OECD countries they are the biggest group of poor families among households with children. Politicians and the media have focused on them as a cause of a broader social breakdown. Yet little is known about the causes, consequences and conditions of lone motherhood in the UK and across different societies. This book addresses these often controversial issues.

*Good Enough Mothering?* provides accounts of historical patterns of mothering and ideologies of the family, cross-national comparisons of policies and experiences of lone mothers in developed and developing countries. It analyses recent social policies and legislative changes in family law, the Child Support Act and discourses about the creation of an underclass in Britain and the United States. Seldom a specific focus of feminist study, lone motherhood has generally been considered through studies of divorce, custody and social welfare. This book contributes significantly to both the feminist and social policy literature on lone mothers.

**Elizabeth Bortolaia Silva** is Research Fellow and runs the Gender Analysis and Policy Unit in the School of Sociology and Social Policy, University of Leeds.

# Good Enough Mothering?

Feminist perspectives on lone motherhood

Edited by Elizabeth Bortolaia Silva

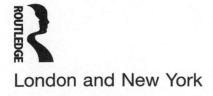

London and New York

First published 1996
by Routledge
11 New Fetter Lane, London EC4P 4EE

Simultaneously published in the USA and Canada
by Routledge
29 West 35th Street, New York, NY 10001

*Routledge is an International Thomson Publishing company*

© 1996 Elizabeth Bortolaia Silva, selection and editorial matter; individual chapters, the contributors

Typeset in Times by Routledge
Printed and bound in Great Britain by
Clays Ltd, St Ives PLC

*British Library Cataloguing in Publication Data*
A catalogue record for this book is available from the British Library

*Library of Congress Cataloguing in Publication Data*
A catalogue record for this book has been requested

ISBN 0–415–12889–7 (hbk)
ISBN 0–415–12890–0 (pbk)

# Contents

# Contributors

**Carolyn Baylies** is a Senior Lecturer in the School of Sociology and Social Policy at the University of Leeds. Her publications include *The History of the Yorkshire Miners, 1881–1918* (Routledge, 1992). Her current research interests are gender and HIV/AIDS in Zambia and Tanzania and the impact of political conditionality on processes of democratization in Zambia.

**Elizabeth Bortolaia Silva** is Research Fellow and runs the Gender Analysis and Policy Unit in the School of Sociology and Social Policy at the University of Leeds. Formerly she taught in the United States at Brown University and at the University of Campinas in Brazil. Her publications include *Refazendo a Fábrica Fordista* (Remaking the Fordist Factory) (Hucitec/Fapesp, São Paulo, 1991). Her current ESRC funded research is on innovation patterns of household technologies and gender relations in households.

**Louie Burghes** is a Senior Research Officer at the Family Policy Studies Centre, in London. Her publications include *Single Lone Mothers: Problems, Prospects and Policies* (FPSC, 1995), *Lone Parenthood and Family Disruption: The Outcomes for Children* (FPSC, 1994), *One-Parent Families: Policy Options for the 1990s* (Joseph Rowntree Foundation, 1993). She is now working on a review of fathers and fatherhood in contemporary Britain.

**Simon Duncan** is Lecturer in the Department of Applied Social Studies, Bradford University, and Associate Fellow of the Gender Institute at the London School of Economics. He is co-author of *Success and Failure in European Housing* (Pergamon, 1994), and co-editor of and contributor to *The Diverse Worlds of European*

*Patriarchy* (Pion, 1994). His current research interests focus on lone mothers and paid work, and on European systems of patriarchy.

**Rosalind Edwards** is a Senior Research Fellow at the Social Sciences Research Centre, South Bank University. Her research interests focus on mothers and education, child care initiatives and lone mother families, as well as feminist and qualitative methodologies. She is author of *Mature Women Students* (Taylor & Francis, 1993), co-author of and contributor to *Mothers and Education: Inside Out?* (Macmillan, 1993), and the *Women's Studies International Forum Special Issue* on 'Women in Families and Households: Qualitative Research', 1995, vol. 18, no. 3).

**Lorraine M. Fox Harding** is a lecturer in Social Policy in the School of Sociology and Social Policy at the University of Leeds. Her books include *Perspectives in Child Care Policy* (Longman, 1991) and *Family, State and Social Policy* (Macmillan, 1996). She has also published various articles on child-care law and policy in Britain. Her current research is on 'family values', fathering patterns and changing gender roles.

**Mary McIntosh** is Senior Lecturer in Sociology at the University of Essex. Her publications include *The Organisation of Crime* (Macmillan, 1975), *The Anti-social Family* (Verso, 1982, with M. Barrett), and *Sex Exposed: Sexuality and the Pornography Debate* (Virago, 1992, editor with L. Segal). Her current research interests are in gender and sexual identities.

**Kirk Mann** is a Senior Lecturer in the School of Sociology and Social Policy at the University of Leeds. He is author of *The Making of an English 'Underclass'?* (Open University Press, 1992) and has written extensively on social divisions and welfare for a number of academic journals.

**Jane Millar** is Professor of Social Policy at the University of Bath. Her main research interests are family and employment change and social security policy. She is the UK representative on the European Commission Observatory on Family Policy. Recent publications include *The Politics of the Family* (Avebury, 1996, editor with Helen Jones), *Lone-Parent Families in the UK* (HMSO, 1991, with Jonathan

Bradshaw) and *Women and Poverty in Britain: The 1990s* (Harvester Wheatsheaf, 1992, editor with Caroline Glendinning).

**Henrietta L. Moore** is Reader in Anthropology and Director of the Gender Institute at the London School of Economics, University of London. She has published extensively on anthropology and feminist theory. She is author of *Feminism and Anthropology* (Polity Press, 1988) and *A Passion for Difference* (Polity Press, 1994).

**Ann Phoenix** is a lecturer in psychology at Birkbeck College, University of London. Her books include *Young Mothers?* (Polity Press, 1991) and *Motherhood: Meanings, Practices, Ideologies* (Sage, 1991, jointly edited with Anne Woollett and Eva Lloyd). She is currently researching the social identities of young Londoners.

**Sasha Roseneil** is University Research Fellow in Sociology at the University of Leeds, where she was previously a lecturer in Sociology. She is author of *Disarming Patriarchy: Feminism and Political Action at Greenham* (Open University Press, 1995), and co-editor, with Gabriele Griffin, Marianne Hester and Shirin Rai, of *Stirring It: Challenges for Feminism* (Taylor & Francis, 1994). She is currently writing a book entitled *Common Women, Uncommon Lives*, which will be published in 1997 by Cassell.

**Carol Smart** is Professor of Sociology at the University of Leeds; she was formerly at the University of Warwick. She is author of *Feminism and the Power of Law* (Routledge, 1989) and *Law, Crime and Sexuality* (Sage, 1995) and editor of *Regulating Motherhood* (Routledge, 1992). She is currently working on an ESRC-funded project on households in transition, which builds on her work on gender and socio-legal studies.

# Introduction

*Elizabeth Bortolaia Silva*

Mothering has long occupied a central place in debates about women's positions in society. Feminist perspectives have asserted that motherhood and mothering are not *natural* for women but that they are historically, culturally and socially constructed. Building on these assumptions, this volume considers recent debates on lone motherhood by focusing on the links between married and unmarried motherhood in historical and cross-national contexts, as well as on policies regarding women's employment, the care of children and ideologies of the family.

The late 1980s and the early 1990s have witnessed an increase in lone motherhood. In Britain, in 1992, there were between one in five and one in six dependent children living in a one-parent family (National Council for One Parent Family, *Annual Report 1993–94*).[1] In the United States it was estimated that by the time they reach the age of eighteen, at least 50 per cent of children and youth will have spent some time in a lone-parent home (American Research Council 1989). Over 90 per cent of lone parents are mothers. Together with this apparently increased 'normality' of lone motherhood, a good deal of disagreement has also emerged over the effects of lone mothering on children, and of the costs of lone motherhood to the budget of the state. The heated debate in Britain in the 1990s stimulated this exploration of the historical roots of the problem, and its comparative national and cultural basis. While the contributors to this volume do not all agree with each other's positions, the contributions offer complementary accounts and point to the difficulties of establishing a fully coherent feminist perspective on mothering in general and on lone mothering in particular.

Lone motherhood has recently been discussed in association with women's independence and gender equality. Do women have the right to pursue careers, to live independently from men and to raise children on their own? Is current public concern an attempt to force women back into the traditional roles of housewife and homemaker 'for the sake of the children'? The politics of gender is at the centre of these debates. The contributions to this book give positive answers to both questions.

The book is structured around three main themes. The first two chapters give a *historical perspective* on mothering and motherhood. The following four chapters address *cross-national comparisons*, with a focus on developing countries and more industrialized economies, particularly richer Commonwealth and European countries. The remaining five chapters focus more directly on the *ideological constructions* that have informed welfare policies addressing lone mothers and their children. The focus is then mainly on Britain, but comparisons with the United States are also made in the last two chapters.

Several issues recur in many of the contributions to this volume.

First, a distinction between motherhood and mothering appears pertinent to interpretations of the changing roles of women both historically and culturally. While a legal connection between mother and child is applicable to motherhood, mothering remains mostly connected to the caring activity *per se*. Although motherhood is not necessarily derived from biology and is a social construction, mothering *per se* is absolutely disconnected from biology. However, there are various connections between motherhood and mothering and very often the terms are used interchangeably. Yet 'good enough mothering' can be well explored as an autonomous feature of various kinds of motherhood (i.e., by adoption, biological, married or lone). The description 'good enough' applies to a mothering that is acceptable, not 'perfect'. It reflects both a diversity in experiences of mothering and the substitutability of the provider of mothering (see Winnicott 1960, 1967).

A second relevant theme is the analysis of links between mothers and lone mothers. On the one hand, they are 'two sides of the same coin'. The constructions of lone motherhood through time and across cultures bear similarities to the constructions of married mother-hood. Women's greater dependency on individual men tends to stigmatize lone motherhood more than in situations where women have greater autonomy. Yet there is no linearity in this process since the achievement of autonomies occurs in contradictory contexts of gains and losses. Also, lone motherhood is increasingly a transient phenomenon, as many women pass through lone motherhood. On the other hand, distinctive features characterize lone motherhood. Poverty and moral stigmatization are recurrent aspects.

A third theme is the distinction between mothers and workers. This relates to ideas of exclusive and sometimes irreconcilable roles for women: either as full-time mothers or working for pay. While full-time mothers require material provision for themselves and their children either from other individuals (usually men) or the state, workers who are mothers of dependent children require adequate child care and guarantees of their ability to provide materially and emotionally for themselves and their children. The scope for choices between the two roles has varied historically and cross-culturally. Feminist discourses have not offered a clear perspective on these kinds of choices. The growing numbers of lone mothers introduce new pressures on the choices involved in these matters.

A fourth feature of many contributions to this book is the presence of cross-national and cross-cultural analyses. They show diverse ways of dealing with similar issues. A very significant comparison is the concept of 'female-headed household' used to identify lone mother families in developing countries and 'lone mother' as applied in developed ones. Whereas the former carries a connotation of responsibility and power, the latter's connotation is of abandonment and loneliness. This is a reflection of both the hardship placed upon women and the agency expected from them, both of which exert particular pressures in developing countries. By comparison, the relative hardship of the lone mother tends to be sheltered in developed countries. State welfare policy regimes and the agencies and strategies of different groups of women are informed by particular 'gendered contracts' regarding the roles of mothers. Ethnicity, religion, class, economic resources and political beliefs play a powerful role in such gender politics and the resulting constructions of lone motherhood and 'adequate' mothering.

Historical transformations of mothering in Britain highlight many of the key general issues regarding motherhood and mothering. As I suggest in Chapter 1, the transformations of 'the mother' are part of the history of women. Conventional histories of women in western cultures have presented the glorification of domestic womanhood and motherhood as a counterpart to both the deterioration of middle-class women's public power and the degradation of working-class women's living conditions as a consequence of industrialization. The acceptance in feminist discourses of these conventional accounts of female historical subordination has led to an implicit and widespread acceptance of the premise of the *degradation of mothering*. The assertion is that either there was a time when mothering was better, or that mothering has been essentially always the same: submitted to by women and controlled by men.

An examination of the 'degradation of mothering' thesis shows that mothering and motherhood have been transformed in contradictory non-linear processes with gains and losses. Positive gains have been achieved by women. For instance, in the late twentieth century the rising lone-motherhood phenomenon reflects changing sexualities in society and increasing autonomy of mothers from fathers. Motherhood and mothering can increasingly be done without men, and women have been able to choose when and how often to bear children. The contrasts with the turn of the century are enormous. However, many continuities also exist, such as the assumptions that still inform the welfare system's allocation of allowances, that mothers are supposed to be dependent on a breadwinner. The change of women from being dependents to providers has been contradictorily interpreted in feminist discourses and is often interpreted as part of a trend towards the deterioration of mothering conditions. The powerful identification of women as mothers inhibits the further development of autonomous mothering.

Historical continuities are given greater emphasis by Carol Smart. Her *revisionist history of motherhood* in Britain (Chapter 2) goes back to the seventeenth century and concentrates mainly on the nineteenth century to consider recent reconstitutions of 'normal' motherhood. She shows that in this period the 'naturalistic chain of events' from conception to motherhood is constructed around the assumption that motherhood is natural. Normative expectations that define what is 'proper' mothering are imposed from this 'natural' base through legal and public policies, aided also by psychological analyses. The legal institution of motherhood prescribes rules that are secured by stigmas and impositions placed upon those who disregard the rules. In the context of 'normalizing motherhood', working-class unmarried mothers are perceived as most disruptive of the norms. They are presumed to be 'bad mothers' in opposition to the married 'good mother'.

Despite the current generalized blame on lone mothers, the recognition that an illegitimate child is not an unwanted child allows for a reconstruction of unmarried motherhood. As divorced mothers came to constitute most of the category of lone mothers, the boundaries of normalization shifted. Yet this also brings a reconstitution of fatherhood aimed at reinforcing men's control of mothering by reinforcing mothers' economic dependence upon men. This is one of the ways in which the reinstatement of the traditional family has been attempted.

Such anxieties about a 'crisis in the family' have appeared in different parts of the world. Henrietta Moore shows in Chapter 3 a recurrent trend of states reducing their own role by pushing more 'social care' into families, or more directly onto women. The implications are that individual women are made responsible for bringing up their children 'properly'. Yet the resources to which women must have access in order to mother adequately are not considered.

The proportion of households headed by women has increased world-wide, redefining women as providers rather than dependents. But this redefinition has many contradictions related to the reasons for women becoming heads of households and the renegotiation of gender roles and expectations in 'families' and in society.

States in poorer countries are seeking to redefine the relationship between the family, the market and the state more profoundly than in developed countries, by portraying the family as an autonomous unit responsible for its own relations with the market. 'Adequate' mothering becomes an impossible task for many. Child labour is needed and many children are abandoned by deprived adults. Turning women into providers without supplying them with adequate resources seems to imply that mothering can be sustained by natural, instinctual provision.

The quality of mothering can be quite irrelevant when the economic viability of mothering is under pressure. This is shown by Carolyn Baylies in Chapter 4 in her analyses of numerous countries, particularly the Zambian example. The diversity in patterns of parenting and household formation world-wide reflects the singularities of colonial experiences of mothering. Norms of the colonialists had important implications for the family structures and kinship of the colonized. Labour migration changed structures of authority, but did not automatically lead to woman-headed households. The varying prevalence of such households is associated with women's access to resources, such as a facilitating legal framework, social tolerance for diversity in family forms, supportive welfare provision, or availability of employment with adequate pay to maintain a household and cover for the costs of children.

Compared to world-wide patterns of lone mothering, the proportion of lone mothers in the United Kingdom appears relatively small (about a quarter of households are female-headed compared to two-thirds in Norway and nearly half in Barbados; see Baylies, Chapter 4). But the problems of lone motherhood loom large if considered from the perspective of British political discourses.

In the UK in the early and mid-1990s, a recurrent argument was that lone motherhood was imposing an unacceptable high cost on society on two fronts. One was the rising social security bill, the other the rising 'culture of dependency' constituted by women wedded to welfare. These social policy problems are explored by Jane Millar in Chapter 5 in relation to the nature of support offered by European and rich Commonwealth welfare states to lone mothers. She finds that welfare states that are most generous to all families are also most generous to lone parents. This implies that benefits tend to be based on women's status as mothers rather than as lone mothers. In this regard, for instance, measures that facilitate the combination of motherhood and employment are applied to all women. The comparison focuses in particular on the Anglo-Saxon and the Scandinavian child-support models. The former tends to enforce financial dependency of individual women upon individual men whereas in the latter the income of the lone mother does not depend on the actions of the separated father. Even so, however, particular features of lone motherhood still recur: lone mothers are at greater risk of poverty than other mothers.

The observation that married and lone mothers have more in common than apart is also examined by Rosalind Edwards and Simon Duncan in Chapter 6. They offer a complementary angle to the assertion by Millar that gender, rather than family status, is the key to understanding the situation of lone mothers.

They argue that a specific focus on lone mothers is essential. For instance, poverty and state-benefit dependency for lone mothers are greater in Britain than in any other European countries. This seems to be linked to low levels of employment for lone mothers in Britain compared to high and rising levels of employment for married women.

Edwards and Duncan point to the workings of 'gendered moral rationalities' to explain the choices and motivations of lone mothers regarding employment. Their comparison of Britain, Sweden and Germany indicates that moral beliefs about mothers – and lone mothers – in paid employment, and the moral acceptance of substitute mothering, are crucial for the uptake of paid work and for claims for the provision of material conditions for the undertaking of paid work. Mothers in Britain are implicitly dependent on a male breadwinner, in contrast to Sweden, for instance, where they are regarded, like all other adult women and men, as workers. The implication is that the moral force to provide for mothers is greater when there is no assumption that there should be an individual male breadwinner to depend on.

However, dependency on the state as an alternative to dependency on an individual man is also highly problematic for women. In the field of social policy this has been a particularly contested terrain for British women since the 1991 Child Support Act. Lorraine Fox Harding argues, in Chapter 7, that the Act represents an attempt by the state to transfer parental responsibility, defined in terms of financial contributions, away from the state. This transfer involves making individual biological parents pay for the costs of children and increases state control and surveillance of pay. Further consequences are that middle-class parents benefit more than those on means-tested benefits, few lone-mother families have benefited, and further problems have been created for second families of absent fathers pursued for maintenance.

These problems of British social policy, and the interpretation that private patriarchy is being restored, could be interpreted as an example of the 'degradation of mothering'. Yet attempts made by the state in this direction have only marginally succeeded, largely because offsetting material and ideological transformations of mothering have led to popular acceptance of lone motherhood as a *quasi-normal* occurrence, in contrast to the discourses of politicians and the media stigmatizing lone motherhood.

A particularly important dimension of the discourses 'demonizing' lone mothers is that they also highlight many problems about dual parenting: rising divorce rates, women's reluctance to marry, women's almost exclusive responsibility for children, and the absence of other alternatives for parenting. Mary McIntosh pursues this line of argument in Chapter 8 to assert that the anxiety about the crisis of the family centred on lone motherhood expresses 'two sides of the same coin'. She exposes dangerous fantasies such as that married mothers' confident dependence on their husbands is more deserving than the lone mothers' dependence on state benefits. If individuals and families should be able to care for themselves, it is vital to recognize that this is not always possible for everyone.

The demonization of lone mothers is particularly strong in relation to the adequacy of their mothering. In Britain the idea of a 'dependency culture' implies the creation of a chain of benefit scroungers. Lone mothering is bad mothering since it is assumed that the traditional heterosexual two-parent family is a better agency for the proper socialization of children. However, the experience of children of lone mothers compared to those in 'intact' families is not as sharp a contrast as the stigmatizing discourses wish. Louie Burghes explores in Chapter 9 the complex, contentious and controversial issues regarding such comparisons of outcomes for children. Increasing numbers of children are experiencing life in a diversity of families and family structures, and children do not have uniform responses to this. The effects of family disruption on children and of lone motherhood may be less important than parental unemployment, poor health, or inadequate education. While difficult transitions in family situations may affect children's outcomes, lone motherhood *per se* does not. These considerations become even more important when it is impossible to assume that families stay stable forever.

The processes by which discourses elaborate demonization include focusing on 'problems'. Thus, those faring well within the stigmatized category are ignored. This is why particular blame has been placed on teenage single mothers by politicians and the media in Britain. Ann Phoenix discusses in Chapter 10 both the construction of teenage single motherhood as the epitome of the problematic mother, and the silence on 'race' in recent moral panics about lone motherhood. Discourses on teenage single motherhood appear as a 'generalization from extreme examples'. The absence of discourse on black lone motherhood is not necessarily positive. It reflects a 'silent discourse'. While black families have consistently been constructed as problematic both in Britain and in the United States, black lone mothers in Britain have not been a focus in discourses. In the USA, lone motherhood has been racialized and this has informed the 'underclass' debate. Yet its absence in Britain does not reflect 'deracialization'. Phoenix suggests that an implicit racialization exists. This intersects with the construction of 'people with a different culture' as the outsiders in the British nation. In this light, the discourses on black and white lone mothers do not converge, as the former are a threat from outside while the latter are a threat from within. Black families are excluded from the ideological construction of Britishness, even as an 'underclass'.

The rhetoric on 'race' has not been translated from the United States to Britain. But anxieties over a 'dangerous and growing underclass' and a feminist backlash linked to lone motherhood have both been prominent in both countries. Sasha Roseneil and Kirk Mann (Chapter 11) discuss these issues, focusing on the claims by 'underclass' theoreticians that solutions to child delinquency are to be found in the reconstitution of the nuclear family and the reassertion of the power and the role of the father within it. They suggest that these attempts at patriarchal reconstruction show a reversal of constructions of dominant power relations, as lone mothers and feminists are pictured as defining the features of society in powerful ways.

The discourses addressing the perils of lone motherhood in the 1990s, as discussed by Roseneil and Mann, show remarkable continuities with the past. For example, beliefs in the civilizing powers of women over men are reminiscent of ideologies of the 1910s and 1920s. In Chapter 1, I show that similar notions supported an ideology of full-time motherhood and made women's employment appear to be a hindrance to the development of proper male responsibilities. Also, gendered role models of the 1950s, which linked inadequate mothering to delinquency (discussed by Smart in Chapter 2), have been reinstated by the underclass theoreticians in the 1990s. The naturalness of mothering, deconstructed by Smart, is also reinstated by the contemporary presumption that mothers instinctually foster morality.

Traditional and conservative ideas still dominate assessments of 'good mothering'. This book contributes to a discussion of these ideas and, it is hoped, to the eradication of many of the worst of them.

NOTE

1    During the second week of December 1992 all of the Queen of England's six grandchildren were living with lone-mother families (McKendrick, n.d.).

# Chapter 1

# The transformation of mothering

*Elizabeth Bortolaia Silva*

The power of women in shaping human beings is central to nearly all conceptions of mothering. In the Judaeo-Christian conception, the woman alone devotedly, unselfishly and wisely gives herself to the task of reproducing new generations. Regardless of her own personal needs, socio-economic conditions or husband/partner, the mother must always subject herself to the ideal.

These views are very familiar. But what sort of mothering do these ideas produce? For some writers of both conservative and feminist perspectives, women hand on misery to women and humanity through their mothering.[1] Yet women also hand on joy to women, and to humanity, through mothering. As individuals, women appear trapped between misery and joy, between full-time motherhood and the rejection of motherhood.

More diverse and flexible views of mothering have existed and do exist. Redefinition, recognition and the transformation of 'the mother' are part of the history of women. And the history of women in western cultures has been structured around very powerful twin stories. One refers to the separation of the public and private sphere, the other to the consequences of capitalism. Put together, the glorification of domestic womanhood and motherhood has been presented in these stories as historically linked to both the deterioration of middle-class women's public power and the degradation of working women's living conditions as a consequence of industrialization.

I argue in this chapter that the view that the present status of women has deteriorated from a past golden age, when they had greater status and an authentic productive function, has had a strong influence on how motherhood and mothering are currently conceptualized. Interpretations of the historical transformation of mothering in feminist discourses have adopted the dominant accounts of women's history and accepted the implicit premise of the *degradation of mothering*. They assume that mothering has been progressively socially devalued, and that there was a time when 'mothering was better', or, alternatively, that mothering has always been essentially the same: with women subjected to it and controlled by men.

The thesis of the degradation of mothering is part of the socialist tradition. It builds on earlier work on conditions of women's work (Clark 1919; Pinchbeck 1930), on interpretations of the rise of the 'cult of domesticity' (Hall 1979, 1980), and more generally on labour-process theory of the 1970s and 1980s. For instance, Braverman (1974) developed a powerful and influential analysis of the 'degradation of work' in capitalist societies. This was embedded in a nostalgic view of a pre-capitalist past when workers had control and autonomy over their labour.[2] For Braverman the essence of the degradation of work lay in the loss of workers' control of the process and product of their labour due to the separation of conception and execution. The parallel thesis of the degradation of mothering emphasizes the increasing subordination of mothers' practices to the prescription of male experts' rules and male-designed welfare policies, with the consequent loss of mothers' autonomy, power and control of their own mothering.

This chapter discusses the theoretical and empirical assumptions of the thesis of 'the degradation of mothering' and focuses on a historical analysis of major changes in Britain since the turn of the twentieth century, particularly in employment, sexuality and child care, to highlight both transformations and continuities. It also discusses the implications of romanticizing the past and examines the implications of the uncoupling of mothering and the 'female' for feminists.

The chapter concentrates on Anglo-American literature and the history of the white middle and working classes. The accounts of the transformation of mothering are therefore limited to this particular western context. Although many trends and relationships analysed here also appear in other societies, an analysis of mothering in France, China, Egypt or Brazil would involve different issues and connections. Yet the general thesis of 'the degradation of mothering' could appropriately be explored in various historical contexts.

## THE DEGRADATION OF MOTHERING?

People are made by other people and bodies are necessary in order for people to be made. This is a universal truth. But the extent to which different people and bodies are involved in this making and the significance of such involvement differ widely.

While mothering has changed historically, there is a powerful continuity in matters of gestation, infant dependence, and the emotional and physical development of infants (Ruddick 1980: note 14). Yet these continuous elements have been perceived in changing ways in different political, technological and socio-economic contexts.

For example, people are born from women's bodies. Yet, not always and everywhere does this turn women automatically into mothers. Solinger (1994) shows that in the United States in the 1950s, white unmarried women who gave birth were positively regarded as non-mothers if they gave the child for adoption. Similarly, since the 1980s, with the advent of new reproductive technologies, women have given birth to 'other people's' children after gestating artificially implanted fertilized eggs (Stanworth 1987) and have not been regarded as mothers. Reproductive technologies have increasingly challenged the social construction of biological motherhood. A woman paid to gestate and give birth to a child for another woman who supplied the egg but who cannot go through a pregnancy herself may not be regarded as a 'biological mother'. On the other hand, a woman who is unable to produce her own eggs but has another woman's egg – donated or purchased – implanted into her womb may be regarded as a 'biological mother'.

However, the biological ties of women and the children they bear have very often and almost universally given rise to the status of motherhood. In virtually all societies, motherhood is an institution with social recognition, rules and legal status. But motherhood can be given up. Mothering can either be attached to motherhood, shared between the mother and other persons, or done in the place of the mother. Motherhood is female, mothering need not be.

A framework that distinguishes between motherhood and mothering is helpful because each refers to a basic set of issues despite their common basis and intermeshed elements. I understand mothering to be a more useful concept for an analysis of historical changes in women's social relationships to children as it widens the definition of a mother to encompass the active endeavour of caring labour.

Why has mothering been so closely identified with motherhood? They have both been associated with women in the context of a persistent male domination of society. In discussions of the degradation of mothering this is generally linked to two major concerns: men's increasing capacity to control mothering, and the progressive devaluation of mothering.

A number of influential analyses of historical developments connected to motherhood and mothering in the United States and Britain (Block 1978; Hall 1979, 1980; Cowan 1983; Ferguson 1983, 1989; Perry 1991) assume that women have been marginalized with modern capitalism. This conviction that 'things ain't what they used to be' has been repeated in women's history (Vickery 1993).

The argument is that when home and workplace occupied the same space women made a substantial contribution to the family enterprise. Then, some time between the late seventeenth century and the early nineteenth century, diligent middle-class women metamorphosed into idle parasites and hard-working poorer women were burdened with more and more tasks under greater male social surveillance and control. Both middle- and working-class women became secluded in isolated homes, increasingly doing as they were told. In the twentieth century the middle-class mother also became 'proletarianized' (Cowan 1983; Rothman 1994).

Feminist analyses have relied on these narratives of the saga of the *bon vieux temps* and 'their sorry demise' for historical accounts of social and economic change in women's lives (Vickery 1993). This conventional explanation of female subordination has important implications for views of mothering as an increasingly devalued activity within capitalism and patriarchy. But such narratives need to be questioned.

These ideas rest on a particular interpretation of the past. For instance, Ferguson (1983, 1989; cf. Block 1978 and Perry 1991) has proposed three historical phases in developments in mothering in the United States. In the first period (1620–1799) women had very little power over mothering because of the identification of motherhood as a natural consequence of the female body saturated with evil lust. Patriarchs held authority to control sinful desires and affections privately and collectively. In the second period (1799–1890) a new ideology of motherhood appeared combined with the cult of domesticity. Motherhood thus became a 'moral vocation' requiring specialized skills. In the third period (1890s onwards) motherhood became devalued. New tasks emerged, and new definitions of standards in child care and housekeeping were set by male experts. Women also became wage workers, and working mothers became overburdened by employment and housewifery/motherhood.

How accurate is this narrative? What are the implications of such assumptions and interpretations?

Similar assumptions are shared by many different writers but are set in rather different chronologies. The 'key historical moment' for the declining role of women as workers and as mothers – or the turning point when a pre-capitalist utopia ceased to exist – ranges from the seventeenth century for Clark (1919), Hall (1980) and Ferguson (1983, 1989) to the early nineteenth century for Cowan (1983). Ferguson (1983, 1989), Block (1978) and Perry (1991) demarcate a period of a rising role for women as 'moral mothers' and argue a strong thesis of the subsequent 'degradation of mothering'. There is a powerful implication of nostalgia for the past. Such a nostalgia is shared even by accounts that place the missed golden past in different chronologies, particularly in the assertion that in much earlier periods women had more status in the household. For instance, Cowan (1983) argues that there has not been a period of high status for the housewife and mother since industrialization began. Hall's period of the 'moral ideology of mothers' is placed within an overall trend of women's marginalization within capitalism (Hall 1979, 1980) (see Table 1.1).

Moreover, to assume, as Ferguson, Block and Perry do, that the

Table 1.1 The accounts of women's marginalization

|  | Declining role | Rising role | Degradation |
|---|---|---|---|
| A. Clark (1919) | late 17th C. |  |  |
| I. Pinchbeck (1930) | 1790 and 1840 |  |  |
| R. Block (1978) | 18th C. (USA) | 1785–1815 | —— |
| C. Hall (1979, 1980) | 17th C. (England) | 1780–1820 esp. from 1850 | since 17th C. |
| R. Cowan (1983) | early 19th C. (USA) | since early 19th C. | —— |
| A. Ferguson (1983, 1989) | 1620–1799 (USA) | 1799–1890 esp. 1840s | 1890s |
| R. Perry (1991) | 1750s (England) | late 18th C. | —— |

ideology of mothering created around the cult of domesticity was a period of women's empowerment seems misplaced. For Hall and Davidoff, the cult of domesticity in the eighteenth century continued to be based upon a rigid sexual division of labour splitting men from women. The space that women controlled – the private sphere – remained wholly subordinate to men (Hall 1979, 1980; Davidoff and Hall 1987). The redefinition of the position of women in the family, upon which 'moral motherhood' was based, was clearly conservative. If material conditions enabled some women to forego employment and willingly dedicate themselves to mothering, paid employment was still important for many others. Women's control over reproduction was largely confined to the middle class. The ideal of domesticity was based upon the role of women assisting men and this pattern continued into the twentieth century.

Have the problems involved in motherhood and mothering worsened since a presumed egalitarian pre-serpent Eden time?[3] Does the degradation trend continue? What have been the more recent characteristics of the 'degradation of mothering'?


## NOT ALWAYS THE SAME

In contrast to the views of a continuing degradation of mothering, discussed in the previous section, an examination of mothering in this century shows how diverse the history of motherhood and mothering has been for different groups of women, particularly the married and the unmarried, the middle class and the working class. By concentrating on the period since the beginning of the twentieth century in Britain, this section examines the relationship between socio-economic conditions and transformations in mothering over time. The focus is on sexuality, employment and child care.[4] The choice of these aspects reflects the concerns of the historical analyses discussed above. Motherhood and mothering are linked in those analyses to social modes of organizing and controlling sexuality, affectionate interactions, and parenting relationships. Since these modes are strongly moulded by mothers' roles in work and labour, the section also focuses on employment.[5]


### Motherhood, sexuality, reproduction and mothering

Historically, we see non-linear shifts of control and autonomy in motherhood and mothering. Despite many arguments about the degradation of mothering, it does not seem that women's control of reproduction and sexuality is today less than it was at the turn of the century. There is a need for more adequate assessments of control and autonomy within feminist discourses. Rather than treating changes in terms of devaluation, my proposal is to focus on contradictory non-linear processes in which gains and losses appear, and where positive gains in control of women's reproduction, sexualities and mothering can also be considered.

At the beginning of the twentieth century, powerful social pressures dictated that women should expect to have children and that they should only have them within marriage. Marriage and motherhood were supposed to be synonymous, and they were regarded as the best achievements for women of both working and middle classes. An unmarried working-class woman could hardly hope to earn even a subsistence wage, and most middle-class women were likewise forced to marry for a living. Although, in general, the centre of the married woman's world was her children and husband (Lewis 1984: 3), the experience of being a woman differed according to the realities of class and bodily experience (Giles 1995: 2). Having time to read books and paying a nurse to look after her child or children was quite different from having to do the laundry while her children tugged at her skirt.

In keeping with the established need for a woman to have a man to keep her and her child or children, legal and social norms were that lone mothers, whether widows, deserted wives or unmarried, ought to keep themselves (Lewis 1984: 56). However, there was ambiguity within state welfare policies on how to treat such women: as mothers or as workers? The most common solution was to take a woman with children but without a man into the workhouse instead of providing her with conditions to earn her own living (Lewis 1984: 62). The granting of outdoor relief was accompanied by greater social control, with deductions being made for 'improper' behaviour (Thane 1978).

Lone mothers were grouped together in these matters, but unmarried mothers were a special focus. Their behaviour was considered immoral and bastardy laws were harsh. Lewis (1984: 11) argues that these laws expressed the state's desire to reaffirm moral values, particularly regarding female sexuality, as well as to curtail social expenditures on this group.

The options for the single pregnant woman were few. In the late nineteenth century, many kept their condition secret or committed infanticide (Horn 1990: 156–7). Some single mothers were assumed to be insane (Spensky 1992: 108). Before adoption was made legal in 1926, informal adoption was another possibility and some babies were sold through advertisements (Lewis 1984: 64).[6] Humphries and Gordon (1993: 169) found that middle-class mothers advertised in the columns of the *Exchange and Mart* for the adoption of children of 'gentle birth', an aspect that made children more attractive to adoptive parents. Some women, however, dared to undergo conventional disapproval and entered 'bachelor motherhood' as a political statement against the control of women's sexuality (Rover 1970: 132–9). They were a small number, but these feminists' advocacy of 'free unions' as an alternative to marriage had some impact on views of women's subordination in the early twentieth century (Bland 1986).

Women's sexuality was understood as reproduction, so motherhood and mothering were frequently treated in terms of women's and children's health problems. A key problem with marital sex was fear of pregnancy and excessive childbearing.

Fertility rates were high, but falling, especially among the middle class. According to Titmus (1976: 95), the average working-class woman, who married during the 1890s in her teens or early twenties, spent fifteen years in pregnancy and birth, with about ten pregnancies. Humphries and Gordon (1993: 5) show that only five in ten pregnancies would result in surviving children, with three pregnancies ending in miscarriage, and two babies dying during birth or infancy. Middle-class women had on average about three children in the 1900s, but also numerous miscarriages and pre-natal deaths.

Infant mortality was also high. In the peak of the 1890s only about three-quarters of births survived (Caunce and Honeyman 1993: 8; Ross 1993). Government statements often stressed women's responsibilities for high infant-mortality rates. Better mothering, it was argued, would prevent infant mortality. Full-time motherhood was therefore stressed, but policies to allow this were absent. Such an ideal reflected an old concern of segments of the middle classes. Hall (1980) argues that, in the mid-nineteenth century, working-class parental attitudes were seen as decadent and inadequate in face of the Victorian ideology of domesticity. Hypocritically, women workers and servants were lectured on the damage done by neglecting their families and children, and middle-class commentators were shocked by the standards of housewifery of factory operatives. Yet women needed to work as domestic servants or in factories to make a living, and struggled to take good care of their families and homes.

The twentieth century has seen significant shifts in these fundamental parameters of mothering, sexuality and reproduction. By the inter-war years, maternal and infant mortality had declined. So had family size. Mothers' lives were no longer dominated by constant pregnancy and childbirth. Birth control was more effectively practised (Humphries and Gordon 1993). Lewis (1984: 20) remarks that the birth control methods used in the 1950s were already available in the 1870s. Yet access was difficult. Lewis argues, like Humphries and Gordon, that the greater control of fertility towards the middle of this century is possibly related to negotiation of relationships and more closely shared views of both husband and wife regarding their life choices. Ross (1993) maintains that contraception was almost exclusively a woman's issue. She argues that in the 1920s abortion (illegal in Britain until 1967) contributed significantly to the declining birth rate.

The ties between sexuality and reproduction were gradually loosened. But this did not imply more flexible codes of sexual morality. Bland (1986: 141) shows that following the acceptance of sexual desire in women before the First World War, during the war itself, 'there were extraordinary restrictions put on the movements of all women and surveillance of their sexual behaviour'. Women's control of their sexualities only re-emerged as a theme from the late 1960s in the context of more effective and wider availability of contraception and abortion (Walby 1990: 169).

In the late 1940s, conservative familialism also took the form of pronatalist concerns. Fabian social philosophy focused on the mother. Policies to make motherhood attractive, however, were ambivalent. Some created nurseries, play centres and laundries to ease the burden on mothers or to facilitate employment. Others gave free access to contraceptive advice and obstetric improvements, and others even planned for part-time jobs to be made available, or for the introduction of family allowances (see Riley 1983: 155–75).

Given the centrality of the ideology of constant maternal care for children's adequate development, even lone mothers were given allowances to stay at home after the Second World War (Lewis 1992a). (Previously only widows received pensions, introduced in 1925.) Benefits were given, and still are, until the child reaches 16 years of age. Any earnings were, and in 1996 still are, deducted pound for pound above a certain small disregard. Sexual 'fidelity' was, and still is, required. The assumption is that a sexual relationship with a man would make him responsible for keeping the woman and her child or children, and result in a withdrawal of state support.

It has been argued that these allowances and benefits were granted because illegitimacy had increased considerably during the war as a result of social dislocation and death. However, after a brief war-time peak of illegitimate births that reached 7 per cent of live births in 1943 and 10 per cent in 1945, the illegitimacy rate quickly dropped to 5 per cent in 1950, staying fairly constant throughout the 1950s. In 1855, the illegitimacy ratio had been 7.8 per cent (Blaikie 1994: 2). In 1961 the ratio for Britain was still only 5.8 per cent, rising to 9 per cent in 1976 (Lewis 1992a: 45). In the mid-1990s it is almost three times higher. In face of this, the introduction of allowances for lone mothers after the Second World War appears to be linked more to the short-term shock of high rates of war-time illegitimacy and the centrality of the defence of the mother in Fabian philosophy. It was also a necessary element of the new Beveridge system of social insurance based on the breadwinner-dependent model of care (Gardiner 1996).

Personal and family life in the 1950s remained conservative. In the sociological literature of the time the importance of the family as a socializing agency was stressed, and well-defined sex roles for men as breadwinners and women as carers were envisaged as the ideal family arrangement (Parsons and Bales 1956; Willmott and Young 1960). On sex matters, there are indications that women and men did not regard good sex as an important issue in marriage, although fidelity was very important (Lewis 1992a: 48).

Yet views about sex and marriage were changing. Divorce and the breakup of parents and their children became common. In 1950, 7.1 per cent of marriages ended in divorce compared to 1.6 per cent in 1937 (Humphries and Gordon 1992: 219). Lewis (1992a: 50–3) argues that the views of the Royal Commission on Divorce appointed in 1951 reflected post-war anxieties about the family. Housing shortages and the falling age of marriage were seen as the main reasons for increased divorce, but women's 'emancipation' was also a major concern.

Growing rates of divorce and lone motherhood have commonly been associated with greater sexual freedom for women (see Smart, Chapter 2, and Roseneil and Mann, Chapter 11, in this volume). Cohabitation has over time become quite common. While only a tiny proportion of the population cohabited before 1960, in the late 1980s more than 20 per cent of people in their mid-twenties were cohabiting (though cohabitation often precedes marriage, particularly following the birth of a child; Gershuny and Brice 1994).[7]

Rather than simply reflecting changing sexualities in society, however, contemporary lone motherhood appears to be part of a more general continuing process of redefinition of gender identities: the increasing autonomy of mothers from fathers. In this process, while particular constructions have been maintained, motherhood and mothering have been dramatically redefined over the last 100 years. If motherhood still has ideological and legal ties of a more traditional kind, economic, social and technological changes have transformed mothering.

Declining fertility rates have enabled women to increase control over reproductive sexuality and to expand their control over mothering work. There are conflicting interpretations of some of these developments. For instance, Brookes (1986: 166) argues, in her study on reproduction from the mid-nineteenth century to the Second World War, that 'scientific' management of contraception and the birth process led to a devaluation of women's traditional knowledge and skills. Medical expertise led to a decline of women's control over their own bodies and a consequent loss of autonomy (see Ehrenreich and English 1979). Yet, contradicting her own findings, Brookes also shows that women increasingly did make choices about when and how often they would bear children, a finding that is never related to her general assessment of degradation of mothering conditions.

Another aspect relating to autonomy and control is that motherhood and mothering can increasingly be done without men. Non-traditional ways of becoming mothers have gained prominence, notably artificial insemination, the 'one night stand', or adoption. Also larger numbers of women have chosen not to become mothers. The proportion of children (below 16 years old) in the total population of Britain has fallen from one-third in 1901 to one-fifth in the mid-1990s. Fertility rates in Europe have declined from 2.6 births per woman in 1960 to 1.54 in 1990 (OPCS in the *Guardian*, 11 April 1995).

Children's demands are also different. Perhaps the roles of mothers and fathers are diminishing in face of the growing importance of peers, teachers, mass media, television, video games and stories. Yet as Davidoff (1995: 11) remarks, contemporary social and political controversy over the role and responsibilities of family relationships in the 1990s has focused almost exclusively on mothers (and marginally on fathers) despite the existence of so many other 'significant relationships' in children's lives. What is classified as 'significant' is subject to change over time. How does this apply to mothers? How has employment been 'significant' in the social constructions of mothers?

## Working mothers

Full-time motherhood implies that a woman is not required to work for pay, that someone – usually a man or sometimes the state – will provide for her and her child or children. It can also imply that she is barred – by legal means or ideologies – from taking on employment. Alternatively, it can signify that the woman will be doubly burdened by the requirement to conform to the ideal of full-time motherhood while additionally taking on some hours of employment as a secondary activity. In this case, if over time mothers have shifted from being dependants to providers, even if secondary ones, this is sometimes interpreted as a trend to the general deterioration of mothering conditions.[8] However, this implies a very narrow view of mothering, defined simply by labour time. Yet the emotional care involved in mothering may be of a better quality when the job is not done full-time, or when the mother has other interests and is rewarded by them. The balance of advantage for women to be drawn between 'mothering' and 'providing' can be a complex and debatable one, and it needs careful appraisal. How often and in what proportions have mothers mothered full-time, who has done so, and in what conditions? Are there transformations over time and what have been their implications?

Around the turn of the century, male earnings were not sufficient to keep a family, and most working-class women had to work (Ross 1993). Yet this work by women was disparaged by legislators in the belief that working-class men would choose idleness if at all possible. Influential middle-class groups argued that, if women worked, men would not feel the responsibility to keep them and their children (see 'Minutes of Evidence taken before the Royal Commission on the Poor Law', 1910, in Lewis 1984: 51; Hall 1979). Male respectability rested on the ability to keep a dependent wife (Lewis 1984: 46–9). Most women agreed with this view, which was fuelled by debates about the family wage in 1912–13, in which feminists were as divided over support for the claim as they had been in the late nineteenth century (Barrett and McIntosh 1980; Land 1980).

Another influence on married women's employment in the first decades of this century was the infant welfare movement's stress on full-time motherhood. Female employment rates at the turn of the century and in the inter-war years were about 32 per cent, the lowest since the middle of the nineteenth century (Hakim 1993: Table 1). The 1931 census shows that, while 70 per cent of single women worked, only 10 per cent of married women had full-time employment (Hakim 1979 in Glucksmann 1990: 42). However, these numbers need to be considered with caution because they are gross national official measures. According to Glucksmann (1990), there were vast regional and industrial variations in the proportion of married women who worked. Although there was some adherence to the ideal of full-time motherhood due to social and legal pressures, such as the marriage bar,[9] women had not only long been industrial wage workers but also had a long history of earning supplementary incomes by a variety of means, such as taking in lodgers (Davidoff 1979), washing and sewing in private households, or manufacturing homework alongside full-time work as housewives and mothers.[10] Moreover, many married women had seasonal employment, not entering the census statistics (Glucksmann 1990).

The view that it was ideal for women to stay at home was widespread between the two wars, when new technology improved daily life, with cars and domestic labour-saving devices spreading to middle-class, servantless households. At the same time, women's employment opportunities were enlarged with the establishment of the very new industries that depended on women as consumers: the mass-produced domestic goods (Glucksmann 1990). What accounts for the inter-war and post-war strength of the ideology of full-time motherhood at a time of labour shortages in crucial expanding industries? Was the ideology of full-time motherhood as overwhelmingly dominant as is pictured in the literature?

Despite firm convictions that mothers' first duties were to their families, increasingly fewer women abandoned work after marriage, particularly after the Second World War. And the woman who did this most often was the working-class woman, who had physically hard factory work, not the one who had interesting and responsible work. As Riley (1983: 145) remarks, 'marriage as an alternative "career" to industrial boredom and low pay' has attractions. Yet, despite the ideology to the contrary, more and more women and mothers took on paid employment. For instance, the participation rate of married women aged 25–35 grew from 9.9 per cent in 1921 to 13.8 per cent in

1931 and to 25.2 per cent in 1951 (Glucksmann 1990: 290, note 11). Employment might have grown even faster if it were not for women being segregated into unattractive 'female jobs' and for the powerful impact of pronatalist and Fabian ideas discussed earlier (Hakim 1993; Lewis 1992a).

Mitchell (1975) argues that psychoanalytic theories were exploited in Britain around the time of the Second World War for ideological purposes. Riley (1983: 90), while criticizing Mitchell on the grounds that it is impossible to separate 'the innocence of a theory and the corruption of its deployment', maintains that, despite the conservative character of contemporary psychoanalytic thought, it cannot be held solely responsible for the judgement that mothers should not work, even part-time, or make use of crèches or nurseries.

Three major social trends have dramatically affected women in Britain in the post-war period. First, the proportion of the female labour force not leaving employment after marriage (mostly employed in part-time jobs since 1971) has risen sharply; second, the divorce rate has increased; and third, illegitimacy has risen rapidly. These changes have shifted the social construction of motherhood, particularly because divorce and illegitimacy have resulted in a steady rise of the lone-mother family.

Have these decisions regarding marriage, motherhood and employment been made in a context of increased opportunities for women? Why have women decided to mother without men and outside of marriage? Why have women decided to carry on in paid employment? How significant are the changes in employment patterns?

The growth in women's labour force participation from about 30 per cent of the total workforce in 1950 to around 50 per cent in the early 1990s (Hakim 1993: Table 3) is certainly linked to smaller family sizes and to the concentration of childbearing into the earlier part of adult life (Gershuny and Brice 1994: 44–7), as well as to the greater availability of part-time jobs. In the early twentieth century, women tended not to have formal employment when they had dependent children, but in the 1990s a proportion of about four in five women in their thirties who have children are also employed (Gershuny and Brice 1994: 48). This makes a focus on employment *and* motherhood more than ever central to an analysis of patterns of mothering.

One argument is that married women's desire to work has become a greater motivation for female employment than their husbands' incomes or lack of income (Lewis 1992a; Roberts 1985; Morris

1990). For instance, the 1980s Women and Employment Survey (Martin and Roberts 1984) showed that 85 per cent of employed lone mothers were working from financial necessity, but only 14 per cent of married women reported that they would not be able to manage at all without their jobs. The centrality of working-mother status goes beyond material needs, although it remains crucially important for certain groups of women. Likewise, interest and enthusiasm for paid work seems to be greater among older women and those in better jobs (Roberts 1985; Martin and Roberts 1984).

However, despite women's increased interest in participating in the labour market, a pattern of sexual segregation has persisted throughout the century. The 1992 British Household Panel Survey (Buck *et al.* 1994) indicated that the typical job status for a woman moves between part-time and full-time work, or from self-employment to waged employment, or between employment and unemployment. Women's jobs have remained low paid and low status, apart from a relatively few career women. Lewis shows (1992a: 81) that in 1901 88 per cent of women in employment were in occupations dominated by women, in 1951 there were 86 per cent, and 84 per cent in 1971. However, Hakim (1994) maintains that between 1971 and 1991 a substantial drop in the degree and pattern of occupational segregation has occurred in Britain and other comparable countries, although occupational segregation persists. According to Humphries (1987) and Hakim (1994), the control of women's sexuality has been a prime reason for such segregation. Hakim (1994) argues that better contraception has diminished job segregation after the 1960s because the social control of sexuality was relaxed once the risk of producing illegitimate children decreased. Yet, since illegitimacy has increased in this later period the correlation between sexual control and labour market segregation can only be partial. Women do not only react to social controls but actively make choices.

In the early 1990s, part-time work constituted about half of all female jobs, but there were twice as many women with children in part-time jobs as women with children in full-time jobs (GHS 1994). In Great Britain in 1981, 25 per cent of women with children under 5 had jobs (6 per cent full-time and 18 per cent part-time) and this rose to 43 per cent in 1992 (11 per cent full-time and 31 per cent part-time; GHS 1994).

The growth of women's employment is also connected to two macroeconomic trends. Since the Second World War, relatively secure, full-time, male dominated jobs in manufacturing have been replaced by less secure female-dominated jobs in services. The trend to increased part-time female employment is linked to the growth of service employment in both public and private sectors. The other trend has been called the 'flexibilization' of the labour force. Increasing numbers of employers have sought irregular employment patterns to fit production fluctuations and market opportunities, thus expanding women's jobs (Cousins 1994).

Casual labour also fits into this pattern since industrial flexibility often implies subcontracting. Women, mostly married immigrant women, are extensively involved in homework in Britain in the 1980s and 1990s. This is a continuity with the past. Rowbotham (1994) shows that legislation to control 'sweated labour', as homework was called in the nineteenth century, was linked to concerns to improve the health of mothers, the homeworker *par excellence* then as now. Boris (1989) makes a similar point regarding the United States.

Labour market trends thus appear to fit well with women's subordinate breadwinning role,[11] enabling – or compelling – them to fulfil their family obligations and mothering demands by broken career patterns, flexible hours, and a lack of training, or availability for homework. It is also probable that labour market trends have built on the inadequacies of social arrangements for women's proper career, pay and job security, notably the restricted provision of child care.

What is the significance of these employment trends for mothering?

Social definitions of women have historically been ambiguous about whether to treat women as wives and mothers or as workers. This ambiguity remains regardless of the relative stability in the level of female employment since the 1880s. In terms of full-time equivalents, the increase in female labour force participation was from 31 per cent in 1891 to only 39 per cent in 1991 (Hakim 1994). Yet social definitions of women, as a universal category, have shifted substantially over time. Unmarried women were basically treated as 'surplus' in Victorian times when a woman had her social existence defined in relation to marriage to a man. In the mid-nineteenth century, unmarried women were treated mainly as workers when young. But the marriage bar made a clear distinction between the married woman (wife and mother) and the unmarried woman (worker). In the 1980s and 1990s, marriage, motherhood and employment have more than ever before become intermeshed. Greater numbers who marry and mother have carried on in paid employment, although they may change from full-time to part-time work. Marriage, motherhood and employment have also become unlinked. While greater numbers of women have decided not to marry or to be mothers, also greater numbers have come either to mother but not to marry or to get out of marriage after being mothers.

Does this pattern of development constitute a devaluation of mothering? The ideology of full-time motherhood has been continuously emphasized, albeit with changing stress. Even though many women refused to fit the ideal, the social construction of full-time mothering nevertheless served as a shield for the social neglect of the needs of women as working mothers. Since caring and mothering have been socially constructed as female, the provision of social care is defined in relation to the socially defined needs of women. This implies that women in part-time jobs, whose employment is not regarded as important, are considered not to require public or employer provision (for example, child care) to facilitate their participation in the labour market.

**The care of children**

The low status of mothers in the labour market has therefore been closely related to the limitations of social provisions such as child care. How has child-care provision changed during the twentieth century?

Proponents of the degradation-of-mothering thesis have often argued that improvements that have facilitated child care – from antibiotics to plumbing – have been offset by rising standards of mothering, including greater stress on the emotional aspects of caring, and that the effective burden of child care has been continuously increasing. How accurate is this assumption?

At the turn of the century, unlike the upper classes who had their children fully mothered by 'nurses' and the middle classes who employed nursemaids to do child-minding (Horn 1990: 76–7), working-class child-care arrangements and provision involved kin, neighbours and schools. Grandmothers and other kin were sometimes paid for caring for children, in the same way as child-minders. Some free care in crèches was provided by state elementary schools to prevent absence from work of girls who would otherwise have needed to stay at home to look after babies. Women seemed to prefer child care through their own networks. Lewis (1984: 56) notes that, in the early twentieth century, crèches were abandoned partly because of economic reasons and partly as a result of pressures by the infant welfare movement on mothers to stay at home with their children.

The infant welfare movement emerged as a result of eugenic concern about the quality of the race: an imperial power needed physically strong and visible rulers (Davin 1978). The emergence of this movement did not change the prescribed role of wife and mother but, at least in theory, recognized the importance of the work performed by mothers (Lewis 1984: 82; Ross 1993). Adequate training for women in housework and mothercraft was emphasized. Many middle-class women found a purpose in teaching social maternalism to the poor or worked as health visitors, rejecting older working-class styles and practices of mothering in favour of a new ideal. The prevalent middle-class ideal mother was a clock-watcher, establishing perfect regularity of habits to achieve character formation. Babies were to be toughened up and made independent of their mothers as soon as possible (Humphries and Gordon 1993: 52). However, Ross (1993) asserts that the new ideal of motherhood had a limited impact on working-class mothers both because of their more relaxed attitude to baby care and because of the constraints of their day-to-day lives which led to babies being more integrated into daily living.[12]

The conservative and patronizing crusade to improve baby care in poor households and the movement to make childbirth safer may have had, however, some positive practical impacts: by the late 1930s a baby's chance of survival had increased four times compared with the rate at the turn of the century (Humphries and Gordon 1993: 55). Improvements in housing and health and social care were also responsible for better survival rates. Clearly most working-class mothers resented the patronizing intervention in their mothering but wanted to be helped to better their family's life conditions (Ross 1993).

It has been argued that the atmosphere of regimentation and increasing control during the Second World War led many mothers, of all social classes, to follow dutifully the prescriptions of the mothercraft methods (Humphries and Gordon 1993: 55–6; Riley 1983). Mothers were increasingly doing as they were told by doctors, nurses, health visitors, and mothercraft manuals.[13] Once the war was over, a more relaxed and permissive approach came into vogue. Mothers were told to enjoy their babies and their families and to form close, warm and loving relationships.

Pronatalist concerns following the Second World War focused on the need for 'adequate' mothering as a means to secure social stability. One key to achieve this was, as it had been at the beginning of the century, full-time motherhood (Lewis 1992a: 11, 21; Riley 1983), but these ideas were now also backed up by psychoanalytic (and feminist) thinking concerning child care.[14] Ross (1993) argues that the rights of mothers to receive public resources, advocated in the late 1910s by the Infant Welfare Movement, was a fading idea by the 1930s. Public discourse came to disregard mothers' work, intelligence and effort as a social contribution. By the 1940s, mothering appears as an aspect of feminine self-fulfilment rather than a social function. 'The dominant discourse did not account for mothers' budgeting, feeding, organizing, cleaning, earning money, and structuring neighbourhood and community life' (p. 223).

During the inter-war years, attention to the psychological needs of the child had become part of the duties of mothers. Freud's thinking reached Britain: women who did not find satisfaction in motherhood were in some way abnormal. Bowlby had also developed his theory of maternal deprivation: a child deprived of his or her mother would develop antisocial tendencies.[15] But theories on child development contained conflicting views, particularly between Klein, Bowlby and Winnicott, as to the essential role of mothers. Winnicott (1953) for instance, while agreeing with the idea that maternal deprivation existed, criticized Bowlby for not taking into account the resources that normal children have to cope with the temporary loss of a parent. In Winnicott's work and elsewhere, space existed within the psychoanalytic discourse for an argument against the need for full-time motherhood. However, this discourse did not prevail.

There is a widespread view in academic and, particularly, feminist literature that the psychoanalytic discourse homogeneously favoured full-time motherhood (Riley 1983 is an important exception). But this fails to consider the disagreements within psychoanalysis regarding the influence of mother-love, hatred, the possibilities of substitute mothering and the role of the environment. The dominance of one line of thought at any one time does not indicate that only one development was possible. Moreover, mothers have also been agents, albeit subordinate ones, in the dominance of the ideal of full-time motherhood. Nor did mothers accept all the prescriptions against maternal deprivation. Some reinterpreted them (Ross 1993; Tracey 1993); others followed the prescriptions of constant maternal care for just a short period until they became exhausted or gained confidence in their own ways of doing things (Humphries and Gordon 1993).

Women's participation in the labour market was not supported by policies to ease the burden of domestic labour and child care.

Summerfield (1984) argues that some policy makers believed that it was possible for women to combine some paid work with housewifery and motherhood with no detriment to standards. Lewis cites various government documents from 1947 to 1951 in which part-time work was thought of as an ideal means to ensure the worker–wife–mother role combination for women. Yet the central government soon closed down the nurseries opened during the war. Nationally there were only 700 nurseries in 1953 as compared to 4,000 in 1943 (*Woman Health Officer*, October 1953, in Tracey 1994: 19).

Riley (1983) argues that the closure of nurseries following the Second World War was not mainly driven by theories of maternal deprivation but rather by central government's attempts to transfer the cost of running nurseries to local authorities. But the financing of nurseries has not been a very popular matter with local tax payers.

Currently, the United Kingdom offers virtually no public provision for child care to employed parents.[16] Employers offer very little support (Brannen and Moss 1991). Mothers rely mostly on their social networks, on their local child-minding system and on the private market. This makes flexible working hours a necessity. Many women work evening or night shifts when child care can be taken over by partners or relatives (Martin and Roberts 1984).

Many middle-class professional households prefer to employ nannies for child care. Gregson and Lowe (1994) associate the employment of nannies with an acceptance of a dominant ideology that children are best cared for in the home by a mother or maternal substitute, and to the needs for help beyond 9 a.m. to 5 p.m. that dual-earner households have. However, cost may be a more important consideration, particularly when more than one child is cared for. A nanny's pay is less than half one full-time private nursery school fee and her working hours are longer or more flexible than those of a nursery. While the job description for nannies (virtually all of whom are women) fits with the 'nature' of female jobs and the availability of women in the informal employment sector, the cost of private nurseries is a reflection of the scarcity of such provision and of the lack of public funding and support for child care.

For many lone-mother households, the non-availability of child care is particularly distressing, affecting the mother's employment opportunities and earning capacity and offering no escape from full-time mothering (see Edwards and Duncan, Chapter 6 in this volume). As lone motherhood increases, tensions between the definitions of women as wives, mothers and workers increase (see Millar, Chapter 5 in this volume).

Are women currently more overburdened with child care than they were at the beginning of the century? As mothering was very different, so were children and what they required. Childhood, for instance, was a much shorter period of life; families had a different division of labour and living space. Comparability is therefore very difficult. However, no specific policies to ease the burden to mothers have been implemented in the twentieth century. Changes in mothering activities have basically happened as a consequence of technical improvements in housing, in science, and in other social constructions such as childhood itself (see Smart, Chapter 2 in this volume).

The experience of the transformation of mothering has been different for the working and the middle classes. But there are great continuities relating to both classes. While working-class mothers have done most of their own mothering, middle-class mothers have historically suffered from the disappearance of servants, and therefore have had to do the mothering that nurses and nannies had formerly been paid to do for them. Yet it is still the middle classes who can most afford to buy mothering. Substitute mothering can be hired for activities ranging from the bearing of offspring, wet-nursing,[17] holding, touching, and body maintenance to psychological support and affection provision. Rothman (1994) refers to this process as the 'commodification of children' and the 'proletarianization of motherhood'. These labels imply a deterioration of mothering. Regardless of whether this is correct, these practices involve only a small proportion of the experiences of mothering in contemporary societies.

Apart from the physical work of mothering, however, one has to consider the emotional job. It has been argued that this has been expanded (Ehrenreich and English 1979; Cowan 1983; Ferguson 1983; Rothman 1994). Ross (1986, 1993) has explored this thesis in her study of London's working-class mothers at the turn of the century. She argues that it is wrong to imply that the 'service aspects' of mothering in the past meant that it involved less emotion than it does nowadays. Her thesis is that caring services to provide for sewing, cleaning, nursing and feeding carried in the past more emotional resonance than they do today. This argument raises the importance of an analysis of the transformation of caring for an assessment of the transformation of mothering.

## CHANGING MOTHERINGS

The thesis of the degradation of mothering agues that motherhood is an increasingly devalued activity within capitalism and patriarchy. The continuous process of degradation is loosely defined around three main features:

1 Work has been intensified by the creation of a multitude of new tasks and raised standards of child care.
2 Emphasis has shifted from care for large numbers of children towards higher quality care for fewer children.
3 Women are compelled to undertake waged labour, regardless of mothering, because of the demands of consumer capitalism, the rising costs of children, and the flight of men from commitment.

The implication of this theory of degradation is that women have increasingly lost control over their own lives and their mothering.

My concern has been to explore the current usefulness and accuracy of this thesis. Can the degradation of mothering be observed in twentieth-century Britain? How do the shifts in the key aspects of mothering, sexuality and reproduction, employment and child care relate to the degradation thesis?

In discussing the thesis of the degradation of mothering I have argued that there is no clear 'progress' in women's positions throughout history. The contours of autonomy and submission have shifted and changed while patriarchies have also been reconstructed, though not necessarily strengthened. Thus, I stress that the paradox in views of the 'marginalization of women', or the 'degradation of mothering', is that whenever female autonomies are developed they are simply subsumed into an assumed pattern of recurrent submission. In this context, lone mothering, an increasingly important aspect of motherhood in the late twentieth century, can be seen in very different ways. Does it, for instance, represent an abandonment of women by men or a sustainable alternative of autonomous mothering by women? Clearly, the interpretation follows from how mothering in general is conceptualized.

Since the beginning of the twentieth century, there has been a movement from dependency on marriage for a majority of women, and on motherhood as a 'natural' consequence of marriage, to an increasing choice about whether, when and how often to have children, and of having and keeping them with or without a man. This has not been a linear process. Nor has this process been externally imposed on women. Declining birth rates appear to have resulted primarily from women's own actions, often without knowledge of male partners, rather than from innovation and availability of technological devices (Ross 1993).

There has been no major change in women's employment rates: large numbers of women have always worked for pay (Ross 1993; Hakim 1993). Yet mothers in employment have been an increasingly larger proportion. A pattern of occupational sex segregation has also persisted, albeit with different contours.

Lack of concern for the needs of women who mother has been another continuity. This is a core element in the degradation thesis because the absence of social provision results in a double burden for the large number of mothers who work for pay. Critics of the 'marginalization of women' theory argue that waged labour is an especially harsh imposition upon wives and mothers. Accordingly, there is an unstated assumption that mothers should have the right not to work in paid employment (Ferguson 1983, 1989; Rothman 1994). Hence, they implicitly endorse the ideology of full-time motherhood. If mothers should not work, should child care be available to them? How can criticisms of the neglect of the needs of working mothers be properly voiced when there is also a view that waged/salaried labour itself is an imposition?

The logic of the thesis of the degradation of mothering points to lone mothers as the product of the flight of men (Ferguson 1983, 1989; cf. Brown 1981). This has some resonance and may apply to many cases. But it also relies on the view that motherhood and mothering are increasingly controlled by men, and that women have continuously lost status and autonomy. However, this is a very partial picture and it seems dangerous to consider lone mothers simply as women who were abandoned by men, victims of rejection. Lone mothering is not simply suffered by women (see Edwards and Duncan, Chapter 6 in this volume).

More generally, the assumption of the degradation of mothering presents women as being passively constructed through history. But mothers are, like other agents, active subjects of history, who create cultural meanings and moral values for themselves and for others (Everingham 1994). Moreover, the degradation thesis also assumes that women do not shape culture through their mothering, because mothers simply reinforce dominant values defined by men and public institutions. Responses to this issue vary widely. Should it be resolved by taking mothering away from the world of men (Kittay 1983;

Young 1983), for instance, or by persuading men to do mothering (Held 1983), or by getting mothering away from women (Bart 1983; Allen 1983)?

All these strategies have been explored in the feminist literature and cannot be resolved here. However, the experiences discussed in this chapter do suggest certain conclusions.

First, mothering is not natural. An account of the transformation of mothering over time shows that mothering is contingent, but also that it evolves in non-linear ways. What mothers do while mothering matters strongly because, whether mothers make autonomous choices or fall under the domination of men, they continually recreate mothering and the conditions under which mothering happens. In this regard, I have argued for the need for more adequate assessments of control and autonomy within feminist discourses. Tensions between them are likely to result in contradictory processes of gains and losses.

Second, mothering is a complex and shifting issue that involves much more than mothers and children. It encompasses ideologies, resources, labour markets, technological changes, men, law, choices and obligations. Shifting social constructions of mothering are closely related to the provision of caring, because mothering is defined in relation to the needs of women as defined by society. The de-packaging of marriage, motherhood and employment alters the social construction of mothering and the definition of the need for social provisions of caring.

Third, rather than construct mothering as an essential psychological or moral attribute of women, constructions of mothering are more adequately addressed in a relational context: the dependencies of children and mothers parallel their autonomies from one another. While the agencies of both create the mothering relationship, this is contingent on structural factors. Dependency and autonomy are not just materially created.

One consequence of constructing mothering in a way that is not centred on women, however, is that it may imply women's loss of a particular kind of control. Since core identities are often constructed on the basis of being a mother and doing mothering, such losses may be painful and may involve large numbers of women. Yet the identification of women with the 'essence' of motherhood seems to have brought no gains for women in other spheres of social life. Nostalgic views of mothering risk stressing losses rather than contradictory shifts, gains and redefinitions. They also underestimate change and fail to take sufficient account of the power of women in shaping mothering in ways that suit their own needs and interests.

## ACKNOWLEDGEMENTS

For criticisms, references and suggestions I would like to thank Jean Gardiner, Katrina Honeyman, Carol Smart and Steven Tolliday.

## NOTES

1  The conservative view is illustrated by the debates of the 1980s and 1990s on lone motherhood in the USA and Britain. It has been argued that lone mothers produce delinquent children and that teenage pregnancy is particularly high among girls raised by lone mothers (Murray 1990; Halsey 1991). Some radical feminists have called for a boycott of motherhood on the grounds that it is the main source of oppression, ultimately responsible for women's subordination (Bart 1983; Allen 1983).

2  For criticisms of Braverman's thesis see Burawoy (1985).

3  Dissent among historians has recently increased about the interpretation of both the roles of the separate spheres and the ideology of domesticity. See especially Clark 1992, Vickery 1993 and Wahrman 1993.

4  While I consider class and gender, race and ethnicity have not been fully discussed in the historical literature available for the earlier decades of the century.

5  Such a broad interpretation of women's lives in different situations over time clearly lacks the flexibility or depth to describe fully differences among women. It is also difficult to define what is typical and what forms group identities, such as married mothers and lone mothers, *the* middle-class mother or *the* working-class mother. There are great internal differences within these groups, as well as regional and local diversities. Similarly, the complexity of the state and its contradictory aims, expressed through different agencies and changing over time, cannot be neatly defined. For instance, the state has often wanted women to work as cheap labour *and* to be full-time mothers. While I am aware of the limitations of generalized comments and the availability of information, it is still possible to make at least some tentative generalizations about important developments.

6  A high proportion of unmarried mothers were involved in domestic service and many illegitimate births were linked to frustrated marriage plans (Horn 1990: 156–7).

7  As a demonstration of practice changing discourse, the Church of England has recently ruled that sex outside of marriage is not sinful (*Guardian*, 7 June 1995).

8  Ferguson (1989) sees in the two wage-earner family a displacement of the focus of exploitation of women from husbands to 'capitalist public

patriarchy'. The argument is that women's wage labour is an imposition of consumer capitalism creating a double burden for wives and mothers. As men's flight from commitment has also increased with the rising costs of children, women are pushed into the labour market, being increasingly penalized (see Brown 1981). Rothmann (1994) takes a similar view in what she refers to as the 'proletarianization of motherhood'.

9    In England the marriage bar, by which married women were kept out of formal employment, was introduced in the last quarter of the nineteenth century and in practice lasted for 100 years, being outlawed only in 1971 by the Sex Discrimination Act (Hakim 1994).

10   These strategies may have resulted in some underreporting of female employment, because only in the period 1901–31 the 'normal' proportion of about a quarter of wives and about two-thirds of widows with some 'occupation' (not domestic work) declined to a tenth. In this century, about a third of the work-force was consistently female before the 1960s (Hakim 1993).

11   Although the numbers of women in employment have increased and women's labour force participation is about half of the work-force, this growth is not reflected in full-time equivalents. Women account for only 33 per cent of total work hours and men for 67 per cent (Department of Employment 1988: 614 in Hakim 1993: 109).

12   Mabel Liddiard, the author of *The Mothercraft Manual*, first published in 1923 and reprinted nearly every year until the mid-1950s, recommended that the baby nursery should comprise two rooms. The garden should be the baby's day nursery. Although she recognized that 'some unfortunate people have no garden', she still recommended that 'At any rate, the largest and sunniest room in the house should be given up to the child' (1954 edition: 33). Despite the guidance on do-it-yourself for many of the apparatuses recommended, the working-class family was unable to afford the material. Babies shared in the family life because housing and life schedules demanded so.

13   Truby King was the guru of the mothercraft movement. In 1917 he established the first mothercraft training school in Highgate, North London (Humphries and Gordon 1993: 51). He was very influential well into the 1950s, as the reprints of Liddiard's *Mothercraft Manual* show. Liddiard was one of King's most enthusiastic disciples.

14   See Myrdal and Klein (1956) as an example of post-war feminist thinking. The recommendation was for mothers to leave the labour force to bear and raise children but to re-enter it as soon as their children reached school age.

15   Bowlby's first influential monograph on the subject was entitled *Forty-four Juvenile Thieves: Their Characters and Home-life* (1946), and his claim that maternal deprivation created delinquency was ideologically very powerful.

16   The Equal Opportunities Commission estimated in 1991 that the existing 700,000 child-care places needed to rise to 2 million. Plans for the American company KinderCare to establish in the UK were based on estimates that, compounded with the rising trend of one-parent families,

by the year 2000 80 per cent of new jobs will be for women (*Guardian*, 21 March 1995).

17   In the twentieth century, the practice of wet-nursing was greatly reduced in Britain. In other parts of the world it remained a common alternative to maternal breast-feeding until at least the 1940s. However, wet-nursing was found to be still in use in the late 1980s (Fildes 1988).

# Chapter 2

# Deconstructing motherhood

*Carol Smart*

Motherhood is not a natural condition. It is an institution that *presents* itself as a natural outcome of biologically given gender differences, as a natural consequence of (hetero)sexual activity, and as a natural manifestation of an innate female characteristic, namely the maternal instinct. The existence of an institution of motherhood, as opposed to an acknowledgement that there are simply mothers, is rarely questioned even though the proper qualities of motherhood are often the subject of debate. Motherhood is still largely treated as a given and as a self-evident fact rather than as the possible outcome of specific social processes that have a historical and cultural location which can be mapped. It is interesting that, in a comparable area, historians and, more recently, sociologists have problematized the concept of childhood (James and Prout 1990). While recognizing that there have always been immature adults, the new sociology of childhood now generally understands that childhood is the product of a number of cultural processes and modernist ideas, which have come to define a specific life stage as different from others and as in need of special treatment, education and moral guidance. It is also assumed (at least in recent British culture) that children should behave differently from adults, that children should be protected from the adult world, and that they should exist in a state of considerable dependence upon their parents or immediate family. As a consequence, childhood has a history; it is not a timeless, transcultural phenomenon but something that has changed and is capable of further change and redefinition.

Revisionist histories of childhood have allowed us to loosen the grip of naturalistic assumptions about the capacities and incapacities of children and the relationship between children and adults, and to become aware of the extent to which modern childhood is of our making rather than a natural phenomenon. This process of 'denatur-alization' has occurred elsewhere, for example, in the fields of sexuality (Foucault 1981; Giddens 1992), disease (Sontag 1983), and gender and sexual difference (Butler 1990; Laqueur 1990). Anthropologists like Edholm (1982) have undertaken the same deconstruction of the western notion of the idealized family, revealing that it is a cultural construct and not a naturally occurring unit. Kaplan (1992) has deconstructed media and popular images of motherhood, and Davidoff and Hall (1987) have deconstructed domesticity and traced the rise of the private sphere as well as the location of white, middle-class women therein. But we do not yet seem to have a revisionist history of motherhood *per se*. Perhaps this is because, for all its problems, the concept of motherhood has been too central to much feminist work. This centrality has arisen in two ways. The first is the way in which motherhood has been identified as a source of women's oppression because of the burdens and responsi-bilities of solitary care, the opportunity costs of caring and leaving the work-force, and the association of child care with menial tasks and limited abilities. This has led to a focus on issues of how to improve the conditions of motherhood rather than a more historical approach. The second is the way in which motherhood has been seen as a source of women's strength and uniqueness, a site that is entirely feminine and that draws upon women's special qualities and knowledge. Thus motherhood has been seen in realist terms, which is to say as an actuality from which women draw strength and from which opposi-tional politics can derive. The institution has thus been given a special status by feminists and non-feminists alike, and, while its parts have been critically deconstructed (such as the rise of domesticity),[1] the whole has not been subjected to a social constructionist analysis. So, while there has been much discussion of the social conditions of motherhood (and how these might be improved or radically chan-ged), there has not been much interest in creating a revisionist history, as opposed to a realist history, of motherhood *per se*.

In this chapter, therefore, I want to start to map out some of the elements of such a revisionist history in the full knowledge that this can only be a sketch that ultimately needs much greater elaboration. I shall do this by focusing on two areas of exploration. The first will question the presumption that motherhood is natural. I want to ask this question because I have become increasingly intrigued by the rise of criminal and other legal measures such as those against abortion, infanticide and contraception. Historically speaking there has been such a heavy weight of machinery brought to bear on women to force them into motherhood we must ask why these measures were necessary if motherhood itself was simply a biological process like ageing. The second will explore the rise of specific normative expectations of white, British motherhood in order to see how the boundaries of 'proper' motherhood are patrolled to ensure that, once established, motherhood takes the appropriate course.

These are important questions for contemporary feminism. On the one hand, giving motherhood a history alerts us to the extent to which motherhood has been a politically contested site for centuries (and certainly not just since the rise of feminism). We need to know that abortion rights are not a new 'freedom', but an old resistance to compulsory motherhood regained. We need to know that there were contraceptive methods used in the past that did not entail potentially damaging drugs. We can thus recapture a history in which women were not simply the victims of Nature from which modern science has saved us. On the other hand we need to expose the construction of dominant normative constraints that create certain categories of mothers as bad or inadequate because they are perceived to fail to live up to the ideals of motherhood that are imposed through legal and public policies.

## DECONSTRUCTING NATURE

To begin any deconstruction of motherhood we have to go behind the mother–child relationship, which is where much feminist work starts, in order to focus on the supposedly natural chain of events that gives rise to motherhood in the first place. Standing behind motherhood, in the shadows so to speak, is a chain of events that are presumed to be so natural as to be inevitable, unquestionable and automatic. This chain of events can be depicted as follows:

sexual activity → pregnancy →birth → mothering →motherhood

But if we examine each link in this naturalistic chain we can begin to understand that this process arises from a number of socially ordained behaviours and from the sanctioning and exclusion of other behaviours. I want to suggest that sexual activity does not *naturally* lead to pregnancy, that pregnancy does not *naturally* lead to birth and so on. Rather than the unfolding of nature we can see a channelling of choices and options that are historically and culturally specific. At each stage of this process, decisions are taken that relate to existing values, social conditions and available options. I shall look at each stage in turn.

## Sexual activity

Since the Victorians it has been almost a tenet of common sense that sex leads to pregnancy. But the idea that sexual activity results in pregnancy is a reflection of the way in which sex itself has come to be seen as coterminous with heterosexual intercourse. Once we decentre heterosexual penetration it becomes apparent that one can be very sexually active without risking pregnancy at all. The questions that we need to consider therefore are when and how did sex become reduced to intercourse and why have we come to see all sex as either procreative sex or as (undesirable) perversion?[2] We have only to think of the Victorian hysteria over masturbation to understand that penetrative sex was actively given a dominant place in the hierarchy of sexual practices and that there were rigorous (although unsuccessful) attempts to eradicate other forms. Following Foucault (1981) we can see that reproductive intercourse was actively 'naturalized' in the Victorian period and other forms of sexual activity became defined as unnatural. This construction of perversions, with dire warnings about dangers to health that would ensue from following such practices, was linked to the rise of medical and psychological sciences.

But the pre-eminence of procreative sex predates the nineteenth century. Christian teaching had long held that sodomy and onanism were sins (although not perversions). Given this long-standing privilege accorded to penetrative sex, the question we need to ask is whether women exposed to the risk of pregnancy sought to avoid this outcome? What seems to emerge as an answer to this question is that before the nineteenth century they did, but during the Victorian era women 'lost' their knowledge of contraception. McLaren (1992) and Flandrin (1979) argue that folk knowledges of barrier methods, coitus interruptus, douching, extended breast-feeding and early forms of spermicides existed in Europe in the early modern period. Long before the availability of what we now regard as reliable contraception, certain families were limiting their size effectively. But it would seem that these folk knowledges were 'forgotten' in the nineteenth century. McLaren (1992: 168) argues,

> English upper-class brides of the late eighteenth century, trained to hide any interest in sexuality, warned not to listen to the gossip of

servants and cut off from the larger female community, were probably more ignorant of the workings of their bodies than their grandmothers had ever been.

Working class women suffered too, he suggests, as practices of breast-feeding changed because of the demand for women's labour and because there was medical and ideological pressure on these women to give up breast-feeding early. He suggests,

> It is possible... that the critique of the birth controllers, complementing as it did that of doctors opposed to lengthy breastfeeding, actually undermined working-class confidence in a measure that offered an important margin of protection to both mother and child.
>
> (McLaren 1992: 188)

The margin of protection he refers to is the cultural practice of avoiding intercourse while a mother was breast-feeding since a successive pregnancy would dry up her milk and put her infant at risk. He points out that, as a consequence, although there was a general fall in fertility rates in the nineteenth century in England, the exception to this was the urban poor.

In addition, we have to recognize that the state was ready to prosecute as obscene any published contraceptive information and that, initially at least, both the medical profession and the women's movement argued strongly against the availability of newer forms of contraception (such as rubber condoms). There was therefore a loss of knowledge, an active suppression both of traditional knowledges and of new technologies, which put women at greater risk of pregnancies at a time when alternative non-procreative forms of sexual expression were being pathologized most actively. The suppression of this knowledge can be seen as part of a strategy of establishing the inevitability of the link between heterosex and pregnancy.[3]

## Pregnancy

While knowledge about contraception was systematically suppressed, knowledge of abortion techniques that would interfere with a pregnancy going to term were also increasingly subject to control in the nineteenth century. Although before 1800 it was a common-law offence to abort a foetus after the stage of quickening or ensoulment (after approximately eighty days) it appears that no one was ever convicted of such an offence (Sauer 1978). Thus it was during the nineteenth century that the criminal law was increasingly deployed to stop this practice and, ultimately, to make abortion a crime at any point during a pregnancy. The refusal to differentiate between before and after quickening marked a vital transition in both religious and folk understandings of the meaning of abortion. As McLaren (1992) points out, until this moment it was not unusual for church leaders to regard contraceptive practices as worse than early abortion.

After the introduction of the 1861 Offences Against the Person Act, the focus of criminal law was directed against the pregnant woman whereas before it had been focused on the abortionist. This marked another important shift away from an 'official' understanding of the problems facing women who were unwillingly pregnant to an active criminalization and stigmatization. What were therefore seen as practical remedies to an unwanted condition became redefined as criminal acts deserving harsh punishment.

This 'escape route' from pregnancy was therefore rendered more difficult, and the inevitability of the supposedly natural chain of sex–pregnancy–birth became increasingly inescapable by the end of the nineteenth century. By this time a whole range of sexual acts that were not heterosexual or penetrative had also been criminalized or actively pathologized (for example, the Criminal Law (Amendment) Act 1885, which criminalized all forms of male homosexuality). Contraception was condemned and abortion made a criminal act. One can begin to understand how motherhood became increasingly unavoidable while at the same time being increasingly hailed as women's greatest goal and most natural of vocations. The rise of this pervasive ideology at the same time as the closure of the 'escape routes' is highly significant and I shall return to this point below.

### Birth and mothering

If a woman has failed to avoid unprotected procreative sex and to organize an abortion, one might imagine that the resulting birth would *naturally* make her a mother. But even birth has not always led to mothering as we now understand that concept. Women of the upper classes did not (and still do not) 'mother' their children, a nanny is paid to do this. Indeed until the twentieth century they might not even have suckled their own babies. Birth was not presumed to trigger maternal feelings or, if it did, the maternal feelings were not the same as those that are thought to constitute maternal feeling today

(Badinter 1981). For women of other classes there were other ways of avoiding the practice of mothering. Infanticide was a long-standing practice available to desperate women. The first specific law against infanticide in England and Wales was introduced in 1623. This draconian legislation applied only to unmarried mothers and worked with a presumption of guilt so that the onus was put on a woman to prove that a still-born baby had not been deliberately dispatched. If convicted of this offence she faced capital punishment. It is well known that juries refused to convict women under these circumstances because people were too well aware of the problems facing unsupported mothers under the Poor Law. The technology was also not available to distinguish adequately between those babies who had been suffocated and those born dead or who died of natural causes soon after birth. But, as Sauer (1978) points out, by the end of the nineteenth century in England there was a veritable moral panic over the numbers of dead babies found abandoned, and presumed killed by their mothers. Doctors were increasingly willing to define infant deaths as infanticides and more women were prosecuted. We begin therefore to see a changing moral climate over the killing of new-born infants.[4]

The birth of a child in the nineteenth century did not therefore seem to herald an instant adoption of what we now presume to be an instinctual mothering role, either by upper-class or by poor mothers. Even poor mothers who did not resort to baby farming, abandonment or infanticide were likely to use their older children to care for new additions to the family rather than to do so themselves, because they had to work to support them. Moreover, the kind of physical care such mothers regarded as adequate would today seem like physical neglect. As Davin (1978) has shown, during the nineteenth century there were considerable energies put into 'improving' the care provided to children in working-class homes and mothers were the primary focus of attention in these new public-health measures.

What this brief historical sketch reveals is that women have had various means of avoiding conception, pregnancy and mothering and that, with various degrees of enthusiasm, they have used folk knowledge and alternative systems of 'care'. This allows us to recognize that the naturalistic chain of events that supposedly leads inexorably to motherhood really only became inevitable at the end of the nineteenth century. We can also trace the growth of increasingly centralized methods to stop women escaping from motherhood. These methods have relied heavily on the criminal law until very recently (for example, abortion was only decriminalized in 1967 in England and Wales) and still rely on legal regulation (assisted reproduction techniques, for example, are available only to certain classes of women). Thus, at the end of the last century and for much of this century, we can speak of women being criminalized if they attempted to rely on traditional means of avoiding motherhood. Such a heavily policed system should make us question the extent to which motherhood is 'natural' save in the most banal of senses. But in addition other, more ideological strategies have also been deployed against women, and this brings me to the final element of the naturalistic chain of events.

## Motherhood

I want to suggest that although (obviously) women have always had children, it is only with the rise of late modernity that we see the emergence of the *legal institution* that we now recognize as motherhood. Before the middle of the nineteenth century, women had no legal status or standing as mothers; put simply, motherhood had no legal existence. Although in practice the unmarried mother was held to be responsible for her bastard, the bastard itself was, in law, the child of no one. The married mother, on the other hand, did not even have these pleasures of responsibility except under the governance of her husband. Only fathers, and hence fatherhood, existed in law. The father gave a child his name, his inheritance, his religion, his domicile; in fact everything a child was granted was treated as coming from the father. The mother was significant in that she brought forth the legitimate heirs, but after that she was little more, formally speaking, than a nanny would have been.

Establishing motherhood as a recognized social and legal institution, with similar rights and duties as fatherhood, involved considerable struggle. This struggle came from two main directions. The first was from (middle-class and upper-class) mothers themselves. Starting with proto-feminist campaigns over the custody of children on separation or divorce (for upper-class women; Norton 1982) and campaigns over wife torture that involved allowing poor women to leave their husbands and to take their children under 7 years of age with them (Smart and Brophy 1985), feminists forced onto the public agenda the beginnings of an appreciation of the work of caring and the importance of mother-love for the welfare of children. These feminists were actively engaged in the social construction of motherhood as a recognized institution. They demanded institutional recognition through the law, and they constructed an ideology of motherhood that rendered mothers as caring, vital, central actors in the domestic sphere, as well as persons with an identity and source of special knowledge that was essential to the good rearing of a child. It is therefore important to recognize that the gradual bringing into being of the legal institution of motherhood was in part a result of political struggle by early feminists who were able to use the ideology of motherhood to try to gain more rights in the nascent family law of the day. These changing meanings of motherhood were integral with other well-documented changes in the nineteenth century, such as the increasing separation of public and private spheres and the rise of the middle classes and their waxing influence over dominant values in civil society.

The second source arose from the work of the philanthropic organizations of the nineteenth century (and later social work, health and 'psy' professions (Donzelot 1979; Davin 1978). These organizations sought to *impose* specific standards of motherhood on working-class women through health education, child protection legislation, and various activities associated with poor relief, such as demands for maternity benefits that would have 'strings' attached. These strings might be the requirement for a doctor to attend deliveries, or they might be requirements for mothers to attend clinics with their babies (Clarke *et al.* 1987). In other instances the imposition of the new values and practices of mothering could be more draconian, as with instances of bringing criminal prosecutions against mothers for leaving their children unattended while they went out to work. A whole range of persuasive policies was gradually brought to bear on working-class mothers to alter their mothering practices. These strategies were strongly supported by ideologies of motherhood that expressed the *natural* characteristics of mothers as coinciding with a class-specific, historically located ideal of what a mother should be. It is vitally important to recognize that this ideology was hardly persuasive in and of itself. Some working-class mothers resisted (and still resist) this hegemonic version of ideal motherhood, but a diversity of mothering ideals could hardly thrive under the pressures that were then exerted. The growth of a more centralized state, and thus the ability to create normative standards and to impose them more uniformly, meant that folk knowledges and customs in child-rearing came under sustained pressure. This meant that there was little appreciation of diversity or even of the difficulties faced by working-class mothers. Instead there were discursively created either good mothers or bad mothers.

## NORMALIZING MOTHERHOOD

Once we recognize the possibility of homogenizing motherhood, made feasible by the institutionalization of certain standards as well as the introduction of more centralized strategies of imposition, we can begin to see how Foucault's notion of normalizing discourse applies to motherhood. As ideals of good motherhood became fixed into policies (say, for example, in relation to the feeding of infants) then it became feasible to apply these standards widely through teams of health visitors, doctors, social workers or NSPCC officers.[5] Thus, taking the feeding example, the mother who fed her infant on demand from a tube (Davin 1978) and the mother who fed her infant from her own plate 'too soon' became inadequate mothers. The good mother either breast-fed her infant herself or fed from a special and hygienically prepared bottle every four hours. (Much later, of course, only breast-feeding defined the good mother, and it was deemed that she should feed on demand and never to schedule.) We can think of numerous examples of minute practices that the good mother should follow, of which the bad mother remained, or so it was often assumed, deliberately or wilfully ignorant. These could range from allowing the infant to sleep in the parental bed (bad), to allowing it to sleep in the same room (all right for the first few months only), to failing to provide enough fresh air (bad),[6] to swaddling or not swaddling, and right through to the modern rules on whether to place a baby on its front (bad now although good in the 1970s and 1980s) or its back (good in the 1990s) to sleep. These rules can be seen in Foucaultian terms as the calibrations of good motherhood. Initially they covered mainly physical matters of diet, warmth, immediate environment, and physical development. Later these calibrations were extended to include the immense realm of the psychological care and nurture of the child. Thus the good mother was no longer simply the one who fed and cleansed properly, she would be inadequate if she failed to love *properly* and to express this love in the *correct* fashion. Love, for example, should not be expressed by spoiling the child, but by very precise gestures and attitudes that were geared towards making the child an acceptable citizen. As Spensky (1992) has shown, for some mothers their love was thought to be best expressed by giving up their babies for adoption so that better-placed, married couples could raise them 'properly'. By the 1970s, however, this mother-love was best expressed by wishing to keep such an illegitimate child.

The fact that the content of the calibrated rules of motherhood changes reveals that there is nothing natural in these manifestations of supposedly instinctual behaviour. But equally, the fact that the content changes does not weaken the overall strength of the system of rules. The significance for Foucault of normalizing discourses is the way in which degrees of adherence to the rules are secured by the stigmas and impositions placed upon those who disregard them. Thus we can think in terms of 'tests' that were and are imposed routinely to discover whether mothers meet or fail the standards of motherhood. There are now myriad ways of failing and, as the range of *expertise* on motherhood expands, so there are added new dimensions of success and failure. In the late twentieth century, even middle- and upper-class mothers can fail since the addition of psychological and emotional criteria has broadened and deepened the areas of scrutiny.[7] However the public focus remains largely where it has always been, namely with working-class mothers. It is working-class mothers and, within that group, unmarried mothers (both black and white) who are still most likely to appear to disrupt the carefully calibrated norms of motherhood. That is to say they are the ones who are deemed most likely to fail on the many tests of what makes a good mother. It is therefore important to trace the history of the unwed mother alongside the rise of hegemonic motherhood, since in Foucaultian terms she is vital to the survival of normative motherhood itself. It is the boundary between the unwed mother and the married mother that has, for so long, been presumed to coincide with the boundary between the bad and the good mother.

## PATROLLING THE BOUNDARIES OF MOTHERHOOD

For there to be a normative ideal of motherhood it is perhaps self-evident that there must be those who 'fall' outside the norm. These two are in a symbiotic relationship and, although the boundaries between them are redrawn according to fashions in motherhood, without the one, the other could not have a social existence. But this moving boundary does not shift in one direction; it is multi-faceted. As one element of the boundary might begin to diminish the significance of the difference between the married and the unmarried mother (for example, some psychological discourses on mother–child bonding), others might be reinforcing negative connotations of

unmarried motherhood (as with emphasizing selfishness or irrespon-
sibility in the context of available contraception). The boundary is
therefore not a smooth line, and the ebbs and flows are various.
However, examining which behaviours and which qualities fall outside good motherhood sheds light on the complex policing of
motherhood and how, rather than being an unchanging and natural
condition, it is a highly contrived and historically specific condition.

Mapping all the elements of these boundary changes between good
and bad motherhood is not possible here and so I shall concentrate on
what I regard as the three main discursive strategies affecting
motherhood since the turn of this century. These are sketched out
in Table 2.1.

In this broad sketch I have identified key *moments* in the history of
discursive interventions into motherhood. These are far from
definitive, but they represent the dominant character of these
discourses and policies at specific times. Through this sketch it should
be possible to identify contradictory shifts and emphases and the
emergence of new methods of marginalizing unmarried or disruptive
(bad) motherhood.

If we read across the columns starting at the top, we can see that

*Table 2.1* Three discursive strategies of normative motherhood

|  | *Psychological discourses* | Welfare discourses | *Moral/legal discourses* |
|---|---|---|---|
| 1900s |  | Poor Law (unwed mothers = economic problem) | Rising illegitimacy (unwed mothers = moral problem) |
| 1910s |  | Insurance principle and early welfare state | Endowment of Motherhood principle |
| 1940s/ 50s | Psychological studies of childhood (Bowlby etc.) | Beveridge Report; Affiliation orders | Illegitimacy and adulterous pregnancies |
| 1960s/ 70s | Focus on mothers | Finer Report and one-parent benefits | Availability of contraception and abortion |
| 1990 | Growth of ideology of fatherhood | Child Support Act 1992; punitive focus on one-parent families and unwed mothers | New Reproductive Technologies |

psychological discourses on motherhood are not relevant until the post-war period. Although training and advice manuals on how to rear children were available to mothers for some centuries before this, these could not be called psychological. Psychoanalytic discourses significant to motherhood do start to be influential after the 1920s when Freud's work is translated into English, but we have to wait until the Second World War before a broader, more normative and empirically based psychology starts to identify the mother as central to the emotional and psychological health of children. Until the 1940s then, we shall focus on the two dominant areas of welfare and moral/legal discourses.

The Poor Law in England began in Elizabethan times, and it remained the primary method of dealing with the unsupported poor until the introduction of the insurance principle in 1911 and the eventual creation of a welfare state in 1945. The Poor Law's treatment of unsupported, unmarried mothers fluctuated in severity. At times fathers were required to pay for the child's keep; at other times they were not (Laslett 1977). Typically unsupported mothers were forced to resort to the workhouse where they would be separated from their children and where they suffered great hardship. Such mothers were seen only as an economic burden on the local state and thus the Poor Law also attempted to act as a deterrent to mothers having illegitimate children. This harsh economic climate and inadequate welfare provision have to be read alongside the moral and legal discourses of the period. Throughout the nineteenth century and at the start of the twentieth century, legislation and moral rhetoric failed to support and indeed punished unmarried mothers. Legal policies rendered them desperate and destitute and the criminal law threatened them with prosecution if they abandoned or neglected their babies. By the end of the nineteenth century, illegitimacy had been constructed as a major social problem. The status of the illegitimate child in law was abysmal, having no legal kin and no common law right to support from either its mother or its father (Cretney 1987).

At the turn of the twentieth century therefore, the position of the unmarried mother was precarious unless she had some kind of protector. Victorian moral purity movements had cast her as the fallen woman and interpreted her motherhood as a result of immorality rather than as an outcome of changing structural and employment conditions (Gillis 1979). But interestingly, the economic position of the married mother was not necessarily much better if she left her husband and he refused to support her. She could apply for maintenance if she was deserted or if he was violent towards her, but mechanisms to ensure that she was paid were non-existent. The main difference therefore between the married and unmarried mother was the former's moral and legal status and standing as long as her marriage was intact. We therefore see emerging a 'grey' area between the married mother and the unmarried mother. This was occupied by the separated (and later the divorced) mother. In terms of welfare policy, the once-married mother might be treated almost as badly as the never-married mother. The only real difference between the separated mother and the never-married mother was the legal status of their children. However, the stigma and the material consequences of illegitimacy could be such that it was much preferable to be a separated mother, even if one endured almost the same degree of poverty. The 'plight' of the unmarried mother and the separated or divorced mother therefore operated as a severe warning to the married mother to keep her marriage intact.

After 1911, the Poor Law was supplemented by provision based on the insurance principle. The National Insurance Act marked the beginnings of a shift in the way that married mothers were to be treated in the twentieth century. It marked the beginning of a recognition that motherhood required a financial supplement from the state and an acknowledgement that husbands were not always sufficient providers for mothers and children. The Act gave women the right to a maternity benefit, but this was an entitlement that could only be claimed through an insured husband. This still bound mothers' fate to the vagaries of their husbands' economic status but it also began the system of exclusion of unmarried mothers from a 'respectable' and non-stigmatizing insurance system. Unmarried mothers were left to the mercies of the remaining elements of the Poor Law or to charity at their time of confinement.

During the period from 1910 to 1940, the position of the married mother gradually improved. Grounds for divorce were extended and her right to maintenance on divorce and separation was consolidated (albeit far from perfect). Even so, there was not a clear-cut distinction between the legal treatment of the separated or divorced mother and that of the unmarried mother. Many working-class mothers who left their husbands still had to use the magistrates' courts to try to get maintenance and so were subject to some of the same indignities as the unmarried mother. Going to court at all for domestic matters was seen as shameful, even if the shame was worse for the unmarried mother. This was because cases were heard in open court alongside criminal cases. Their details appeared in local newspapers and so the separated mother, like the unmarried mother, had no privacy for her affairs at all.

At the level of moral rhetoric, a very significant feature of this period was the rise of the campaign for the Endowment of Motherhood. This campaign, which eventually led to the introduction of Family Allowances in 1945, can be seen as one of the most powerful discursive strategies of the period (Macnicol 1980). The writings and lobbying of the Endowment campaigners established the idea that the mother was not only central to the health of the family, but that she should be entitled to an independent financial recognition of this. This was more, therefore, than moral invective. Although success in policy terms was not achieved until after the Second World War, we can witness a gradual recognition of the significance of the institutionalization of motherhood as a basis for new citizenship rights in the form of benefit entitlements.

In 1942 the Beveridge Report was published (Beveridge 1942). It appeared during the Second World War as the promise of a new social order when peace was achieved. It proposed the complete sweeping away of the remnants of the Poor Law and the introduction of an integrated, national system of both insurance-based and means-tested safety net benefits. Beveridge's proposals, including a family allowance, were introduced after the end of the war. In his Report the role of the mother was recognized as vital to the post-war reconstruction. Her role was to be the good wife and fecund mother. The nascent welfare state thus continued the presumption that the married woman would be financially dependent upon her husband; indeed, through its structure of benefits, the new machinery ensured that this would be the case. This meant that the unmarried mother remained highly vulnerable because, although she could insure herself while in work, she would lose benefit rights once she left work to look after her child, including her later pension entitlement. In any case, she was likely to be sacked the minute her pregnancy was discovered since no women then, married or otherwise, had employment protection when they were pregnant.

What is interesting is that these proposals came into being at a time when illegitimacy rates had increased considerably because of the war and there was also an increase in adulterous pregnancies where married women had become pregnant by other men during their husbands' absence (Smart 1996). These changing social conditions were not recognized in the Beveridge proposals, possibly because it was assumed that the end of the war would mean that conjugal reproduction would resume its ascendancy and that, in the new social order, illegitimacy would become marginal.[8] At this stage, one of the main methods of attempting to deter unmarried motherhood and adulterous pregnancies (apart from the lack of financial support) continued to be the punitive and stigmatizing status of illegitimacy that was visited upon the child. Spensky (1992) shows that at this time it was still thought to be far preferable for an unmarried mother (or an adulterous mother) to give her baby up for adoption, whereupon it would be legitimized, than to keep the baby who would have to carry the stain of illegitimacy.

The introduction of the Family Allowance in 1945, payable to the mother rather than the father, gave concrete substance to the enhanced status of motherhood in a general sense. But equally, the important studies by Bowlby (1953) and Winnicott (1957) heralded a new emphasis on the importance of the mother for the emotional health of the child. As Riley (1983) has argued, Bowlby cannot be held directly responsible for the way in which his theories were taken up and applied, but his work on the supposed damaging effect of separating mother and child did give rise to an orthodoxy about the need for mothers to stay by their young children almost constantly. This emphasis on the mother was a mixed blessing. On one hand it meant that it was presumed that mothers would keep the children if there was a divorce or separation, on the other hand it was always mothers who became the focus of blame if children became delinquent or maladjusted. In particular, attempts by middle-class mothers to go to work during their children's formative years and the need of working-class mothers to stay in work to support their families were treated as major crimes against childhood and the stability of the next generation.

It was the dominance of this psychological paradigm that gave rise to the insistence that unmarried mothers should surrender their children for adoption at this time. This shows a remarkable shift in management of illegitimacy from the moral presumption that the child was the punishment for the sin and that the mother should not be relieved of the burden of care to the equally firmly held belief that the mother must give up the child. In the first instance, the concern appears to be that the mother should sin no more. In the second it appears that the concern has shifted to the 'quality' of the child and its ability to grow into a well-adjusted citizen. In neither of these models was the welfare of the mother at all significant.

It took some time before the core idea, that mothers were important to the psychological health of their babies, was extended to include unmarried mothers. Because there was presumed to be a natural bond between a birth mother and her baby, it became difficult to sustain the idea that this was only the case if the mother was legally married. Policy began to change until it came to be assumed that if an unmarried mother did not have a legal termination (available after 1967) then she would keep the baby. This shift came about for several reasons. One crucial element was the realization that an illegitimate child was not, automatically, an unwanted child. In any case, mothers started to refuse to give up their babies. The wider availability of contraception (after 1964) and abortion meant that unwanted babies could more readily be avoided or unwanted pregnancies could be more readily terminated. In addition, the distinction between the unmarried mother and the divorced mother also became more blurred. After the 1960s, the category of lone mothers was predominantly constituted by divorced mothers rather than never-married mothers. It therefore became more difficult to 'brand' all such mothers simply as feckless.

The late 1960s and the 1970s can therefore be identified as a discursive high point in the history of motherhood. In 1974 the Report of the Committee on One Parent Families was published (Finer 1974). The Finer Report made substantial and radical proposals to extend the support offered to lone mothers from the welfare state. Most crucially it proposed to ignore, for benefit purposes, the route by which mothers found themselves caring for children alone. The hierarchy of lone mothers (from widows, to the divorced, to the never married) would have been virtually swept away if the proposals had been adopted. But his ideas were seen as too radical and too expensive and they were never implemented. None the less, for our purposes, the mere existence of such a Committee and such a Report shows how far, discursively speaking, the status of the unmarried mother had been reconstructed. Moreover, during the 1970s there were gradual changes to the status of the illegitimate child such that the distinctions between the legitimate and the illegitimate became less and less significant. In addition, the availability (albeit not universal) of contraception and abortion meant that two of the elements of the inevitable and supposedly natural chain of events between sex and reproduction were diminished. The 1970s therefore gave rise to the possibility of sex without reproduction and, should a woman choose to become pregnant, the decade held forth the promise (if not the actuality) of the possibility of fully autonomous mother-hood. It is during the 1970s that we can see positive shifts towards lone motherhood in all the three discursive fields of psychology, welfare and moral/legal. This was therefore an extremely important moment in the history of motherhood because motherhood stood on the threshold of independence (from the governance of men and marriage) and in sight of a proper means of economic support. However, the promise of this moment did not survive the end of the 1970s.

In the 1980s we can see a number of significant shifts again. I shall outline these below, but first it is important to note that after the 1970s it is the lone mother (whether divorced or never married) who is reconstituted more firmly as a burden on the state, as an inadequate mother to her children and as damaging to the moral fibre of society. Within this category of lone mother, the never married may have been seen as somewhat more culpable, but it is the general category of lone mother that was, once again, demonized. It is in the 1980s that we witness the rise of men's and father's rights movements, which sought to challenge the new status of the lone mother (Smart and Seven-huijsen 1989). These movements sought, on the one hand, to eradicate the husband's financial responsibilities for his former wife and, on the other, to increase his rights in relation to his children (legitimate and illegitimate). Figuratively speaking, we can say that fatherhood emerged out of the shadows again to try to reclaim its lost status in the family and in wider society. These claims were enhanced by a revival of psychological studies that purported to prove the link between the absence of the father and delinquency in the child (Dennis and Erdos 1993), which mirrored to some extent the 1950s and 1960s ideology of motherhood. Thus fatherhood became ac-cepted as being emotionally and psychologically vital for the welfare of the child. This father was not construed as the distant disciplinar-ian or stout economic provider but as an engaged and caring parent. The influence of this movement was such that changes were made to family law so that it was no longer possible for mothers to gain the sole custody of children on divorce.[9] This re-enhancement of fatherhood, along with the continuing demonization of lone mothers as economic burdens on the public purse, led to another legal change. This was the introduction of the Child Support Act in 1991. This measure was designed to recoup benefits paid to lone mothers from the biological fathers of their children. This measure threatened fathers with the same sort of financial penury that previous laws had imposed on unwed mothers and divorcing mothers prior to the 1970s (see Fox Harding, Chapter 7 in this volume). In this respect we can see the Child Support Act as a means of bolstering marriage through economic measures and thus, indirectly, as a way of trying to reduce the incidence and the costs of lone motherhood.

This renewed antipathy towards the lone mother could be found elsewhere in the 1980s (see also McIntosh, and Roseneil and Mann, Chapter 11 in this volume). The growth of reproductive technologies such as *in vitro* fertilization (IVF), as well as the more mundane practice of artificial insemination, came under scrutiny. While these practices raised wide ethical concerns, a subset of concern was focused on the unmarried and widowed woman who might want to become a mother through the use of such techniques. The 1990 Human Fertilisation and Embryology Act limited the access of unmarried women to these procedures and imposed an indelible mark of illegitimacy on any child born to a widow using her husband's gametes posthumously. Thus we can see that, with the rise of new technologies, new distinctions were drawn to preserve the boundaries of good mothering.

## CONCLUSION

In terms of these prominent discourses of motherhood it is possible to argue that it was in the decade of the 1970s that the boundaries between good and bad motherhood were most blurred. Not only were there increasing material supports for different forms of motherhood, but alternative household organizations were prefigured and motherhood began (symbolically and to a lesser extent actually) to escape the normative constraints of psychological and moral orthodoxy. Legal and policy changes also made it possible for motherhood to detach itself from the governance of the father. But this brief moment (for now it would seem that it was quite fleeting) has been followed by a renewed discursive closure for the possibilities of motherhood even though the actual number of lone mothers keeps rising. The reconstitution of fatherhood has had important consequences for motherhood because it has not been a radical reconstruction of men's responsibilities so much as an attempt to demote the significance of the mother who was thought to have become too powerful in the 1970s. We can speak of an ideological attempt to reprivatize motherhood, by which I mean an attempt to reinforce mothers' economic dependence upon men at a time when other avenues of economic independence for women continue to be limited. There is, in the 1990s, a renewed fear of the consequences of allowing lone motherhood to thrive positively as opposed to by default. Morgan (1995) for example, has argued that not only does lone motherhood lead to delinquency and other maladjustments, but that women's independence from men will produce a new 'warrior class' of young men who have no attachment to their communities and no responsibilities to keep them law-abiding. Married, dependent motherhood is seen as a means of civilizing men who otherwise return to a supposed state of nature. Such arguments seem to be gaining ground and the lone mother is once again depicted as the source of almost all social ills. Yet such views seem to be completely devoid of a historical perspective on motherhood and family life prior to those that occurred in Britain in the 1950s. In particular, it ignores the extent to which the 'traditional family' was a nineteenth-century construction that was dependent upon clear strategies of disempowering women and binding them to motherhood and the private sphere in a way that was unprecedented. This is not to argue that there was once Utopia, but merely to stress that what is now an idealized form of motherhood was the product of certain historical developments. It is increasingly important to sustain a knowledge of the history of motherhood in the face of this new orthodoxy. The revisionist history I have outlined here can only be a small part of such a project and is itself, of course, a contested 'version' of events. I am conscious, for example, that this history is an institutional history and not a history of women's agency and resistance. But this history at least suggests that women have not always fallen into motherhood as if it were simply their destiny. Moreover, we can see quite clearly how motherhood has always been a site of contested meanings and values. Given this history, we should hardly be surprised that motherhood is again on the political agenda in Britain in the 1990s.

## ACKNOWLEDGEMENTS

I am grateful to Lorraine Harding, Kirk Mann, Elizabeth Silva and Pippa Stevens for comments on an earlier draft of this chapter.

## NOTES

1 One should not forget the pioneering work of Sally McIntyre (1976) on the ideology of motherhood and the response of the medical profession to pregnancy in married and unmarried women.

2 These are questions that radical feminism has been asking for some time of course.

3 I use the term 'strategy' in the Foucaultian sense, in that I do not presume that there was a specific group of people or of interests that devised this strategy with a clearly articulated purpose or aim.

4 This was mirrored in the measures introduced to control baby farming and to end the practice of allowing parents to insure the lives of their infants. Both of these practices were seen as ways of, or as encouragements to, the snuffing out of infant life. The first involved mothers sending their children to minders for up to a year. During that period they would not see the child and it was highly likely that the child would die, especially if the rates of pay were low. The policy of allowing parents to 'benefit' financially from the death of an infant was stopped because it was believed that it simply encouraged poor mothers to allow their children to die.

5 As Beatrice and Sydney Webb stated in 1910, 'In the ignorance and listlessness, and absence of standards, which characterise whole sections of slum-dwelling families, there was... the very minimum of fulfilment of parental responsibility .... It is the watchful influence by inspection and visitation, advice and instruction, brought to bear on the mother... that evokes the sense of responsibility, guides and assists its fulfilment, imposes the higher obligations of rising standards... in the working class mother of the present day.' (See Clarke et al. 1987: 67.)

6 Both of these requirements could be very difficult for working-class parents who might only have one room, or who could only afford to heat one room and so on. Anna Martin, writing in Common Cause in 1911, notes that 'If a baby is to survive, Harley Street tells us, it must have plenty of air and space, abundant mother's milk or satisfactory substitute, regular hours for food and sleep, and exercise. All these the typical Hampstead baby has, none of these are available for the average Bermondsey one.' See Clarke et al. (1987: 68).

7 It might, for example, now be argued that the Queen was not a good mother to Charles because she was so distant and because she sent him to boarding school.

8 In fact illegitimacy rates did fall considerably in the 1950s, but began to rise again a decade later.

9 The Children Act 1989.

# Chapter 3

# Mothering and social responsibilities in a cross-cultural perspective[1]

*Henrietta L. Moore*

Mothering and motherhood are not, contrary to popular belief, 'the most natural things in the world'. They have taken very different forms in different times and places. What it is to be a 'mother' is both cross-culturally and historically variable. Historians writing about wet-nursing and child fostering in Europe remind us how very different motherhood was in the past, and how little it resembled the project of a full-time, home-bound, isolated career on which the ideal of Euro-American motherhood has been based in this century (Pollock 1983; Aries 1973; Lewis 1986). Recent work has also emphasized the degree to which the experiences of mothering, and of being a mother, differ according to divisions of race and class (Glenn *et al.* 1994; Cock 1980; Hansen 1989, 1992; Thornton Dill 1988). Women working as domestics might relieve their employers of some of the heavier burdens of motherhood, but this left them very little time to attend to their own children or for the maintenance of broader family relationships. Mothering and motherhood thus vary within specific contexts as well as between them.

Motherhood and the context in which it is supposed to operate, 'the family', have always been sites of contestation. The state has a clear interest in intervening in the production and reproduction of the work-force, in the delineation of units of welfare provision and taxation, and in the structuring and maintenance of differentiated social identities (Moore 1994a; Molyneux 1985; Abramovitz 1983; Barrett 1980; Stacey 1983). This is particularly clear in colonial contexts, where the social construction of mothering was part of a larger project of societal reconstruction involving the management of social and racial differences (Jolly and Macintyre 1989). In many cases, failure to conform to standards of idealized mothering led to stigmatization and discrimination.

Ideologies of mothering and motherhood necessarily exert considerable influence and pressure in all situations, but the degree to which they determine practice is very variable. Dominant ideologies of mothering and motherhood certainly coexist alongside subdominant ones, but those who do not or cannot conform to the dominant ideologies may pay a heavy price. Recent debates about mothering and lone parents in the UK and the USA demonstrate this point since those women who have apparently demonstrated their inability to mother within a 'complete' family have paid with social stigmatization and cuts in welfare provision. The issues here are many and complex, but tend to revolve around whether mothers can be workers, whether women who have children should be able to support them, and whether those who parent outside of a conventional nuclear family should expect support from the state. The rhetoric that has animated this debate has inevitably drawn on ideas and assumptions about the role of women, about what constitutes adequate mothering and about the 'natural' form of the family. The impact of the debate, however, has not been confined to the USA and the UK, but has extended into the international arena and formed part of a larger discussion about the relationship between the family and the market, the role of the state in mediating that relationship, and the problem of how to limit rising welfare costs. This discussion has been fuelled not only by pragmatic or financial concerns but also by the often rapid social changes that many countries and communities are experiencing. Globalization and market integration, coupled with other factors, have had an uneven but none the less dramatic impact on family structures and household livelihood strategies. The result in many cases has been a general perception of disequilibrium and unsought-for change in family life. The validity of and reasons for this perception are difficult to judge, and would require specific analysis in each context. It would certainly be more than foolish to make global generalizations, but it is the case that anxieties about a 'crisis in the family' have found fertile ground in many places, albeit for rather different reasons.

## THE FEMINIZATION OF POVERTY

One major recent change in family/household structure that has attracted much comment has been the reported rise in the proportion of households headed by women. The reasons for this increase, like its rate and magnitude, are diverse, but it is a trend that has been noted for many different countries in the world at varying patterns of economic development.

It is evident that the number of female-headed households is related to marriage strategies, property and inheritance transfers, as well as the intersection between production systems and the repro- duction of labour. This means that it is unwise to treat female headship as a unitary phenomenon. The definition of headship itself complicates the picture because of the variable relationship between economic provision, decision making and structures of power and authority. Women, for example, are rarely classified as heads even when they are the major economic providers if there is a male over 15 years in the household, while men are frequently designated as the head even when they are not the major provider.

One significant cause of the rise in female-headed households in developing countries is labour migration.[2] Out-migration is on the increase as disparities between rural and urban locations, and between countries, become more marked. While significant and growing numbers of women migrate, the general growth in migration figures is reflected in the number of women left to care for children and maintain household reproduction without the help of a spouse. However, it is important to distinguish between those households where male labour migration has resulted in female headship and those where women are involved in polygynous marriage or have been abandoned, divorced, separated or widowed. It is equally crucial to note that many households will pass through a phase of female headship during their developmental cycle, which may be because of migration or because of divorce and subsequent remarriage or because of a subsequent marriage by the husband. The analysis of female headship thus needs to be closely tied to an examination of life cycles, marital strategies and labour deployment.

A recent study of family welfare in Ghana disaggregated the available data and looked at different types of female-headed house- hold. Households headed by married women were found to be best off and those headed by widows worst, with the households of divorced women in an intermediate position. However, it is the case that larger households containing adults of both sexes have improved access to cash income as well as lower dependency ratios.[3] It is also evident that women's overall access to income and labour is improved through co- residence with men, particularly spouses, because women suffer discrimination with regard to their access to land, capital, education and credit.

On average, the study found that female-headed households in Ghana are no worse off than male-headed households and are slightly less likely to be found in the lowest quartile of the income distribution. Thus, an increase in the proportion of female-headed households does not necessarily indicate a growing concentration of poverty among women, but it does suggest their increasing primary economic responsibility and their growing vulnerability. Some women may have no choice except to become a household head – particularly those who are widowed, divorced or become lone mothers when very young – but it should not be assumed that membership of a female-headed household is always a disadvantage for women or necessarily deleterious for child welfare (Lloyd and Gage-Brandon 1993: 118).

Data from the Ghana Living Standards Survey document the critical role played by women's work in all households with resident children. Male household heads do almost no domestic work, even though such work has important productive value. Women work more hours in total than men, but fewer market hours. Women's access to the cash economy makes an important contribution to the economic standing of households with children. The adjusted consumption levels of household members are highest in households where women have a primary work role either as co-head with their husband, or as primary head of their own household.

The straightforward assumption that poverty is always associated with female-headed households is dangerous, both because it leaves the causes and nature of poverty unexamined and because it rests on a prior implication that children will be consistently worse-off in such households because they represent incomplete families. There are a number of points to be made here. First, the overall findings from Ghana are supported by data from elsewhere that suggest that resources under the control of women are more likely to be devoted to children than are resources in the hands of men (Dwyer and Bruce 1988; Haaga and Mason 1987; Kennedy 1992; Buvinic et al. 1992). Thomas (1990) found that income in the hands of Brazilian women increased the health and survival chances of their children, and that it had an effect on child health almost twenty times greater than income controlled by the father. Nutrition data from the Northern Province of Zambia show that children under 5 years old in female-headed households are less likely to be malnourished than children in slightly better-off households where both parents are resident. The reasons for this have to do with women's improved access to child care and to networks of sharing within female-headed households (Moore and

Vaughan 1994). The available data suggest that the income that poorer women earn can lead to higher health and social benefits than the income men earn (World Bank 1993).

To argue that the position of female-headed households is complex and internally differentiated is not to deny the validity of data from around the world that show them to be disadvantaged with respect to property, capital, income and credit. Many such households exist in the context of nation states that are rolling back their boundaries and pushing more 'social care' into the arena of the family. This phenomenon provides a particularly graphic demonstration of the way in which women are expected to carry a disproportionate share of the costs of child care and social reproduction, and to do so often from a diminished resource base. Furthermore, the distribution of the costs of social reproduction – caring for children, the elderly and the sick – are inequitable within family/household units. As Nancy Folbre argues, the distribution of income and labour time within families is an important determinant of economic growth and welfare, and yet it has remained largely unmeasured and unexamined because of the persistent tendency to analyse families as undifferentiated and altruistic units (Folbre 1983, 1986, 1991). In all societies, the family contributes a very large share of the time and money devoted to social reproduction, that is the production and maintenance of 'human capital' (Folbre 1991: 3–4). The unequal distribution of income and labour within the family means that women carry a disproportionate burden of the costs of the reproduction of that capital.

Women's particular responsibility for the reproduction of human capital is often reflected in the way they are held to be primarily responsible for child welfare and for any inter-generational transfer of disadvantage. Much of the recent research on single mothers points out that these women's own lack of resources, including poor education, contributes to increased levels of child mortality and delinquency, and decreasing levels of educational attainment and life opportunity for their children. The easy elision between female heads of households, teenage pregnancies and dysfunctional families works to make these linkages seem obvious and pre-given. Aggregate figures and generalized categories, such as 'teenage mother' and 'lone parent', exacerbate this tendency. Premature parenthood, for example, does appear to be increasing in many developing countries (Population Reference Bureau 1992), and when it is associated with low educational attainment, low rates of marriage, low wages and low levels of property inheritance and transfer, it will also be associated with poverty (Yeboah 1993). But to speak of women in such circumstances as being responsible for the inter-generational transfer of poverty and/or disadvantage to their children is more than disingenuous. For one thing, it implies that the individual is to be held accountable and that she is somehow at fault for not bringing her children up in a 'proper' family. This places the responsibility firmly on the individual for her failure to achieve economic and social security, and effectively prevents a thorough analysis of the causes and consequences of poverty. Teenage pregnancy does not cause poverty, however strongly it may be correlated with it under certain circumstances.

Focusing on women in the case of premature mothers and lone parents reveals the extent to which women are held to be responsible for child welfare in a way in which men are not. In fact, the reported rise in teenage pregnancies in some contexts may indicate that it is the young men who are refusing to marry. The reasons for this are diverse, but perhaps the most significant factor is that under conditions of economic decline, and where family labour cannot contribute directly to production, the cost of children has become too great. This is particularly the case where male employment opportunities and wage levels are also in decline. Increasing numbers of men are finding that they cannot support families and that marriage acts as a net drain on their own meagre resources.[4] Even among middle-class families, it has become evident that some men are using their greater bargaining power within the household to renegotiate the distribution of responsibilities so that women shoulder a greater proportion of the costs of child-rearing and welfare. This means that, where women are able to earn an income, they may find that they are forced to take on the cost of the running of the household, while the husband retains his own income for other purposes (Dwyer and Bruce 1988).

## THE COSTS OF CHILDREN[5]

The overall cost of supporting children is one thing, but from the point of view of family welfare what is important is the distribution of those costs between parents and the pattern of their overall contributions. This section of the chapter examines these issues and argues that women bear a disproportionate share of the costs of child care and socialization, and therefore of the reproduction of human capital. The key question here is 'What are or should be the consequences for policy of recognizing that women shoulder a larger proportion of the costs of reproducing the human capital on which future economic prosperity will depend, and that they do so from a diminishing resource base in many instances?'

The distribution of income and labour time within the family is closely connected to the costs of children. An important determinant of the cost of children is the level of contributions they will make as they mature (Caldwell 1982). These contributions may be in the form of labour time, waged income, remittances and support in old age. The perceived level of these potential contributions influences fertility and decisions about investment (including school fees). However, another important determinant of the cost of children is the contributions that will be made by society as a whole, including health care, education and family allowances. When the levels and nature of both forms of contribution are considered alongside the distribution of the costs of child care between parents, a clear distortion emerges.

Several studies from various countries have shown that mothers work longer hours, consume less and devote more of their resources to their children (Dwyer and Bruce 1988; Sen 1983; Folbre 1986). The commitments that women make to motherhood reduce their earnings, labour market experience, promotional prospects and general potential for economic independence (Folbre 1991). Women, as mentioned earlier, carry a disproportionate share of the costs of child-rearing and the reproduction of human capital. But do they recoup those costs in particular ways? It has been argued that under certain conditions of production and reproduction in the developing world, with a strict division of labour and defined cultural expectations, women are partially recompensed in two ways. First, regulations governing kinship and marriage clearly set out men's responsibilities to dependants. Second, women can expect economic contributions from their children (Nugent 1985; Cain 1982).

But, as Folbre (1991) argues, increases in the cost of children due to processes of modernization and market integration have intensified the economic stresses on families. The rising costs of family life have intensified conjugal conflict and negotiation, rendering women in some contexts even more vulnerable in consequence of the unequal distribution of power in conjugal unions. This augments the probability of individuals reneging on formalized contracts, such as marriage, and on informal contracts, such as expectations of support for kin, elderly parents and other household members. Children and the elderly are increasingly unable to participate in a wage-based economy, where education is crucial, and they become more vulnerable to poverty. In this situation, parenting becomes a commitment with many costs and potentially few rewards. Each case must be analysed in specific terms, but what is evident is that in these sorts of circumstance women are no longer receiving any recompense – or very little – for the disproportionate costs of child-rearing and nurturing that they bear.

It is not possible to make global generalizations about family structure, family law and welfare policy. But transfers (pensions, family allowances) are often structured to provide benefits to waged employees and to reinforce a family structure based on a male breadwinner (Folbre 1991). The result is that social security pro-grammes discriminate against female wage earners despite attempts in many countries to reform the law (Brocas *et al.* 1990), and they do so in a situation where women are already discriminated against in the labour market. Part of the explanation lies in the fact that levels of family benefits are quite low in relation to other public transfers. Working women pay the same level of taxes as men and thus contribute equally to total public transfers, but the proportion of such transfers reallocated to family benefits is relatively small in a situation where women are still bearing a disproportionate share of the costs of child care. Benefit levels and welfare legislation vary enormously around the world, but women who are raising families on their own are not receiving sufficient support compared to families with a male breadwinner. A review of current social insurance programmes in Latin America and the Caribbean concluded that such programmes subsidize children in families headed by full-time wage earners, effectively redistributing money away from most families maintained by women alone (Folbre 1994). Female-headed households might represent a significant proportion of the state's welfare bill in some contexts, but this is not because they are dysfunctional families, but because they are bearing the full costs of child-rearing and nurturing in systems where public transfers do not adequately address the fact that all women shoulder a dispropor-tionate share of the burden of social reproduction.

## FATHERS, HUSBANDS AND CONJUGAL EXPECTATIONS

Certain critics of welfare policy have argued that welfare programmes provide perverse incentives and increase marital dissolution. As Nancy Folbre (1991) points out, economic development and fertility decline have historically been accompanied by increases in the percentage of female-headed households and by institutional changes that redistribute some of the costs of social reproduction from families to society as a whole. Welfare programmes then are the result of these changes and not the cause of them, and there is no evidence to suggest that providing benefits to families increases marital instability. Critics sometimes argue that welfare programmes are a form of unproductive spending, but this is rarely more than a way of arguing that the cost of welfare provision is too high. It is evident, however, that women's ability to support their families, whether they are married or not, would be greatly enhanced by improving their position in the labour market and instituting education and training programmes. Such an initiative would also have benefits for child health, nutrition and education. Family programmes should really be treated as employment programmes in the widest sense.

It is an irony of the fact that women do shoulder a disproportionate share of the costs of child care and human capital reproduction that debates about female-headed households inevitably focus on why women end up in this situation. The implication is that the women themselves are responsible for an increase in marital instability and that this may be connected to growing numbers of women in waged work and/or to changes in role expectations and attitudes. Relatively little attention, as mentioned above, is given to fathers and to the role of men in changes in family structures and gender role expectations, even though quite a lot of research has been done in this area.

## Women and waged work

The question of whether women's involvement in waged work leads to an increased sense of independence, as well as improved decision-making roles in the household and changes in conjugal role expectations, is impossible to answer in comparative perspective. The empirical findings have been mixed, and it is difficult to know, for example, whether women divorce because they have the ability to be self-supporting or whether they enter the labour market when they recognize that their marriage is unsatisfactory. Recent data from Thailand, where women have a long history of employment and where the divorce rate is low but showing a modest rise, suggest that what little effect employment has is mediated by a whole set of factors relating to marital problems, wife abuse and poor relations between spouses. The picture is further complicated by the fact that 25 per cent of families in Bangkok are extended, and hence women may have help with domestic duties and child care. Some women keep a shop at home or are craft workers and they can therefore integrate domestic and productive work more readily. The study concludes, however, by pointing out that, although work might allow women to leave an unsatisfactory marriage, it certainly does not cause divorce (Edwards *et al.* 1992).

Divorce rates are on the rise in many countries of the world, but it is worth noting that this pattern is not a uniform one and that in many countries women are unable to divorce. There are also marked differences between rural and urban areas, and between individuals of different classes, religions and ethnic groups. The available data suggest that women suffer a significant loss of income at divorce, with reductions of 30–70 per cent from pre-divorce family income, while men's income tends to increase because they are no longer supporting dependants (Weitzman 1985, and see the discussion of Lloyd's and Gage-Brandon's material above). The result is that divorce and marital disruption have very different consequences for women and for men. The reasons for increasing divorce rates have to be specified culturally and historically, and no single generalization could cover all the kinship and marital systems of the world. However, a number of critics have asserted that rising divorce rates are related to changing roles and expectations, and that, among many factors, increasing female participation in the labour force, greater mobility and modernization are to blame. These arguments are difficult to assess – especially in comparative perspective – because they are often based on assumptions about the negative effects of social change on what are thought to be key social relations and cultural values. What is evident is that critics frequently approach the problem of changing roles and expectations within marriages and families from an individual as opposed to structural perspective.

Recent research in the South African homeland of Qwaqwa has produced evidence of high rates of premarital pregnancies, conjugal conflict and marital dissolution, accompanied by poor socialization of young males and rising levels of crime (Niehaus 1994; Sharpe 1994; Banks 1994; Moore 1994a). The reasons for this situation are a decline in male migrant labour and male employment generally, increasing social differentiation within the community and the relocation of industries (clothing, glass and electronics) into the area to take advantage of cheap female labour and other incentives. The consequence of these changes is that household reproduction is more dependent on female income from beer brewing, petty trade and waged labour. Women report their husbands as saying that beer brewing is not an appropriate activity for respectable married women, and that domestic tasks and child care are being neglected as a result of women working. Conjugal conflict over income and household decision making has been greatly exacerbated as men transfer their anxieties about the loss of their jobs and their declining contribution to household resources into the domestic domain. Women find themselves increasingly in the position of not being able to support the family on a male wage and they continue to look for ways to generate income. There have been a number of violent clashes in the homeland where men have protested against the provision of jobs for women in the new industries at their expense as they see it. Conjugal roles and expectations are being forced to change, as women provide more of the income while partners are unemployed. Child care, especially for women with young children, has become a crucial issue. The definitions of a 'good wife' and a 'good husband' are altering, and one result is that people's personal relationships are under enormous pressure.

The forms and structures of families and households are responding to these changes in a number of ways. The dependency ratios of adult income earners to children are a clear determinant of household security among low-income households, and consequently extended households made up of three generations or co-resident siblings are emerging. Increasing numbers of women are refusing to marry because marriage provides little security for them and their children, while increasing their vulnerability through the demands that husbands can make on wives' labour, time and income. More and more men are leaving the area and not returning because they cannot support their families. Young men are refusing to marry and/or to acknowledge paternity because they do not have the resources, and are not sure that they will ever have the resources, to enter into family commitments. As mentioned earlier, marriage in this kind of situation becomes a net drain on men's resources and this is one factor involved in the increasing numbers of absent fathers and unmarried teenage mothers.

Under conditions of extreme economic and social pressure, it becomes apparent that women's and men's interests do not converge but rather diverge. The needs, rights and obligations on which the conjugal contract depends can no longer be mutually constructed. This should not, however, be taken as straightforward evidence of the breakdown or dissolution of the family. Co-residence of adult, unmarried siblings was noted by Niehaus (1994), who reported sisters who went out to work and had their children looked after by their brothers. Family ties between generations were strong and a number of residential arrangements involving grandparents and grandchildren and multi-generational households were noted. Family ties of a broader kind were actually essential for establishing wider networks and residential arrangements that would allow households to secure access to income and to nurture the young. In the past, many analysts have failed to recognize this point because they have been implicitly comparing such family arrangements with the conjugal, nuclear family, and have thus found them wanting.

The question of crime, especially among young males, is clearly related to the high levels of unemployment and to the impossibility of establishing adult status in a situation where you can neither marry nor work. The need for an income in order to be able to consume and survive is what draws some men into co-residence with their sisters and others into illegal methods of income generation. There are no incentives for young men and very few opportunities for creating a positive sense of self. It is not so much that fathers are absent and have no authority, thus providing defective role models, but rather that the whole structure of masculine identity is in doubt. This may in turn provide further impetus for involvement in illegal activities that bring their own form of status, recognition and identity. The problem of unsocialized youth is but one part of a larger problem about the care and nurturing of the young.

## CHILDREN IN THE LABOUR FORCE AND ON THE STREET

We cannot understand changes in the ideologies and practices of mothering and motherhood without recognizing that such changes must be connected to changes in the nature and experience of childhood. Anthropologists and historians have long pointed to the culturally and historically variable nature of childhood. The different conditions of children's lives generate different definitions of childhood, and individual children's subjective experiences of childhood will vary according to the specific understandings and ideals prevalent in any one context. The roles and tasks of children around the world differ, as do views about what is reasonable to expect from a child. This becomes particularly apparent when we look at children in the labour force, and the related problem of children on the street.

Unicef estimates that around the world over 100 million children work, and this figure does not include farm and domestic workers. Twenty-five per cent of children between the ages of 6 and 11 in low-income countries are working and not in school, and of those between the ages of 12 and 16, approximately 60 per cent are working. Over 100 million school-aged children receive no education and over 100 million children live on the street. About 150 million children in the world are malnourished (Unicef 1990). In India, it has been estimated that 22 per cent of male working children start full-time jobs at 8 years or younger, and another 25 per cent by the age of 10. Girls start their working lives earlier, either as maidservants in middle-class households or as housekeepers and care-givers to younger children in their own household. Those in the latter category are surrogate mothers and not remunerated. Over 50 per cent of employed girls receive no cash payment for their work, while only 7 per cent of boys are unpaid. Where girls do receive payment, 96 per cent hand over all their salary to the family, as compared to 52 per cent of working boys (Schlachter 1993).

Two things keep these children working: the economic necessity of parents and the economic advantage of employers. The two are connected. Low levels of wages in the informal and formal sectors of the economy for the urban poor, and especially for adult women, make child labour a necessity in order to bring in enough income to support the family. As the need for an educated work-force grows, children who have been pulled out of school to work, particularly girls who start to substitute for their mothers very young, will be at a particular disadvantage in the labour market. Employers find child labour attractive because children are paid less than adults, they are easier to control and lay off, and they are unable to insist on their rights.

The large numbers of working children in urban environments are related to the problem of children on the street. The available data show that children are on the street in increasing numbers, and it is often assumed that these children are without families and involved in crime and drugs. Recent work on children in urban environments has emphasized the importance of distinguishing between children who simply work on the streets and those who may be working on the streets but are without families or homes.

Among homeless working children, there are different degrees of connection to the family and of marginalization. Some visit their families frequently, preferring to live closer to their place of work with other children, while others do not have the money to travel home. There are also children who have run away or been abandoned. A recent five-country (Kenya, Brazil, Philippines, Italy and India) study by Unicef found that these children had often left home to avoid cruel treatment by a parent or step-parent or because the family had suffered a tragedy such as a parent's death (Szanton Blanc 1994). The heavy obligation of bringing in money, combined with strict parental control and beatings for the slightest misdemeanour, led many children to flee home. Sometimes such children were lured away from home by another child who could point out the advantages of being independent of parental interference and not having to work under impossible conditions to help support younger siblings. Children from female-headed households were not significantly more likely to be among the homeless, but dislike of step-parents who failed to provide support and affection in return for the child's contribution to home life was an important factor for many children. In the case of Brazil and Kenya, households that were notionally female headed often had resident adult males in them, compounding the difficulty of correlating female headship with child homelessness. What the study did find was that poverty was the major factor forcing children into work, often at as young as 6 years, and that being in work and being very poor provided the context in which children were forced away from their families. Most of the homeless children interviewed, albeit in the rather different contexts provided by the five countries, expressed a great deal of sadness at having moved away from their families and retained a strong sense of the family as a potentially supportive and loving unit. Many of them had left home because of a lack of support and affection, not surprising in the context of poor families where both parents are working very long hours themselves for very little money.

Children on the streets are vulnerable to exploitation from adults and they are easily drawn into prostitution, drug, alcohol and solvent abuse, gambling and crime. Children are exposed to rough-handling and sometimes brutal treatment by security guards and the police. In Brazil, the killing of street children has been attributed to various so-called 'justice committees' said to be made up of off-duty policemen and security guards (Swift 1993), and there have been reports from Colombia of shopkeepers and other civilians killing homeless children and child beggars (Buchanan 1994). Children often move around in gangs, which give some protection and offer a sense of belonging and commitment. The Unicef report on Italy pointed out that children who cannot acquire prestige, recognition and a sense of self at home or in school are particularly vulnerable to the lure of participation in petty crime, gambling, stealing handbags and motor scooters, and handling drugs. There is a strong sense of self at work in being able to manage the hostile urban environment and escape control and/or detection by adults and the authorities. The net result is that children often identify strongly with the violence they experience and subsequently engage in violence themselves (Lorenzo 1993).

Prostitution is a common way to make money for boys and girls. In Nairobi, where strong links between the street children have been observed, girls may be selling sexual services during the day and returning to their 'community' at night. These alternative communities or families may involve pairing between girls and boys who consider themselves 'husbands' and 'wives'. However, sexually transmitted diseases are a major health problem. A recent study in Brazil reported that street children engaged in sexual activity with peers and adults from inside and outside their circle. Sex was a means of acquiring money, food, clothes or shelter, but within the peer group it was used for entertainment, pleasure and comfort, as well as to exert power and establish dominance. Of the children interviewed, 42.9 per cent reported having sex under the influence of drugs or alcohol, 39.4 per cent had sexually transmitted diseases, 69 per cent of girls said their friends had been pregnant, 43.4 per cent that their friends had had abortions and 60 per cent of boys reported experience of anal intercourse. Sexual initiation occurred at an early age: averages of 10.8 years for boys and 12.4 years for girls. Many of the sexual encounters street youths described were exploitative or coercive, and girls were particularly vulnerable to sexual violence and exploitation. The findings revealed that street youths were more vulnerable than children living at home to sexually transmitted diseases, including HIV/AIDS, and that street girls were more likely to get pregnant and/ or have an abortion (Raffaelli et al. 1993).

Once children are on the street they are vulnerable in all sorts of ways, and this applies whether children are genuinely homeless or not, although those who are homeless are even more vulnerable. Children on the street are particularly vulnerable to exploitation by adults. The inculcation of some into a 'culture' of violence, petty crime and substance abuse reflects the harshness and brutality of their circumstances, as well as the necessity to make ends meet. These children do suffer from emotional deprivation and from a brutal reduction in their life chances, primarily because of their lack of education. However, there is very little direct evidence to suggest that the plight of these children is the result of incomplete or dysfunctional families. Poverty and low wage levels force families into a situation where they must substitute or augment adult labour with child labour, and once that process is established the route to a street existence becomes possible.

## THE SITUATION OF MOTHERS AND CHILDREN

Nation states in the developed world are finding the cost of welfare programmes hard to meet, and are alarmed by the speed and scale with which these costs are projected to rise. In this context, the debate about the family is one of the mechanisms through which states are seeking to redefine the relationship between the family, the market and the state. This process of redefinition is crucially dependent on portraying the family as an autonomous unit that is responsible for its own relations with the market. If a family fails to provide for its members then this failure is an individual one and may be attributed to a lack of effort or to the dysfunctional nature of the family unit. There has been an increasing tendency to blame women as wives for the failures of marriage and women as mothers for the misfortunes that befall their children. However, the material presented in the previous sections cannot be explained as the result of inadequate mothering or marital dissolution. Families are under pressure.

However, many women are under very specific kinds of pressure. Research shows that women shoulder a disproportionate share of the costs of child care and the reproduction of human capital, and the disadvantage of female-headed households provides graphic evidence of this fact. Women receive no compensation from either the market or the state for the burden they carry. The inability of female-headed households to manage in some contexts is a result not of the fact that they are dysfunctional families but of the discrimination that women suffer in the labour market and of the unequal distribution of labour and income within families.

The supposed indicators of 'family crisis', marital conflict, youth crime, disadvantaged children and lone mothers are not the result of 'dysfunctional' families, and must also be seen in the context of the strain placed on certain family relations and categories of individuals by poverty and extreme economic hardship. Lack of control over their lives forces many disadvantaged families into situations where personal relations breakdown under stress. Loss of self-esteem both for parents and for children, combined with joblessness, unwanted pregnancies, substance abuse and despair, is made worse by the fact that poverty also dispossesses people of their political as well as their economic rights. Those who are not employed and have little education are very unlikely to have much say in the conditions of their citizenship and/or in political processes in their countries.

The increasing tendency to blame families, and very often women within those families, for their inability to survive the structural changes wrought by increasing market integration and globalization is one way of avoiding an analysis of the causes and consequences of poverty and immiseration. Progressive market integration has led to increasing differentiation both between and within countries. What is more alarming is that processes of social and economic differentiation have intensified along lines of gender, race and class (and other forms of difference) with potentially disastrous effects for certain groups within populations.

Women shoulder a disproportionate share of the costs of raising children and they therefore carry a disproportionate share of the costs of the reproduction of human capital, of those who will support us all in the next generation, the labour force of the future. Investing in children, in their education, security and health, means investing now in their mothers. It means recognizing that mothering and motherhood are diverse practices that necessarily respond to variable family/ household structures and strategies. They are not natural categories or activities, but complex means of providing children with emotional and material support. The available research suggests that increasing the health, education and welfare of women leads to increased benefits for children. It is extremely unlikely that legislation or coercive pressure applied through welfare sanctions will bring down the divorce rate, transform the nature of marriage or increase family stability. The simple recognition of this fact should encourage policy makers to look at ways of improving the welfare of children as part of a strategy to safeguard the productive capacity of the future. Such a strategy will have to be based on supporting the women on whom those children depend.

## NOTES

1 This chapter uses material first published as an UNRISD Discussion Paper for the Social Summit in Copenhagen, 1995 (Moore 1994b).
2 Data from Botswana in the 1980s showed that 42 per cent of urban households and 47.5 per cent of rural households were female headed, and the figures overall suggested both a decline in marriage and an increase in migration for males (Van Driel 1994: 25).
3 Dependency ratios are defined as the number of resident productive adults in a household compared to the number of dependants (children, elderly, sick).
4 Data from Mexico bear out these attitudes by men towards marriage and children in situations of economic stress (Chant 1991), and data from Africa point to the large number of women deserted by male partners once they become pregnant, as well as cases where husbands or partners refuse to contribute to child maintenance (Van Driel 1994: 173–6, 189–203).
5 My argument in this section and those that follow is indebted to the work of Nancy Folbre (1991, 1994) from whom I take my understanding and inspiration.

# Chapter 4

# Diversity in patterns of parenting and household formation

*Carolyn Baylies*

The percentage of single female-parent homes is featured in a table entitled 'weakening social fabric' in the United Nations Development Programme's *Human Development Report 1994*, alongside such other measures of presumed social dissolution as intentional homicides by men, asylum applications received, and juveniles as percentage of total prisoners. Data in the table refer exclusively to industrial countries and the column on single female-parent homes only to OECD countries.[1] While this reflects the dearth of comparable statistics cross-nationally on such measures, the fact that data on households headed by women should be placed under this title at all suggests some curious presumptions about the directions of social change and the nature of idealized norms. Such presumptions, however, belie a diversity of experience, the dimensions of which will be explored in this chapter.

In the UK, the proportion of all families with dependent children headed by a lone parent rose from 8.6 per cent in 1971 to 19.2 per cent in 1991, with the parent being female in nine cases out of ten (Haskey 1994: 7).[2] There are some who see these figures as very much a measure not just of the weakening but of the renting of social fabric, with particular concern being expressed over those regarded as flaunting an aberrant status and scrounging off the state. State policy providing support for lone parents has been criticized as misconceived, far too generous and as contributing both to a decline in marriage and the creation of a 'warrior class' among youth practising predatory sexual behaviour (*Guardian*, 3 January 1995).[3]

Anxiety over increases in lone-parent families, involving not just an appeal against what is believed to be misconceived policy but also worry over a more general post-industrial malaise as the dominance of the nuclear family is perceived to be slipping away, is frequently premised on a particular interpretation of the historical relationship between the family's structure and function on the one hand and economic change on the other. Goode's (1963) attempt in the 1960s to provide a comprehensive, cross-cultural, historical analysis of the family, albeit within the context of modernization theory, acknowledged vast differences in type but also specified certain continuities and commonalities – among them the tendency for industrialization to have as its correlate a transition to the conjugal family, characterized by monogamy, bilateral descent, relatively free choice of partner and the nuclear family household as the normal residential unit for the rearing of children. While much challenged, these generalizations have a strong hold on the collective imagination. Should the conjugal family be posited as characteristic of modernity, at the very pinnacle of the developmental process, then any evidence of its apparent disintegration may assume the basis for disquiet. Thus while all lone mothers may be tarred by the same brush, it is those regarded as voluntarily placing themselves in this category – by having children outside of marriage or being divorced or separated – who are particularly scorned. Such condemnation appears to rest upon the assumption that successful, adequate or 'good' parenting involves parents being married to each other as well as their ensuring proper socialization and the private provision of emotional and financial support for their children. It assumes, moreover, that such support and socialization can only occur where both parents are resident in the same household, despite the questionable elision between parenting, household and family that such logic implies.

Imputed meanings and understandings regarding patterns of parenting and household formation need to be closely examined. In practice, innumerable variations are possible and invariably occur. The presence of two parents in the same residence gives no guarantee of either financial or emotional support, let alone effective socialization, nor that parenting will in fact be a joint, shared enterprise.

The relationship between economic change and family forms also requires careful consideration. In Guadeloupe in the Caribbean, a single parent allowance has excited similar outrage from some quarters to that in the UK, with recipients of state funds having been accused of '... symbolically and in fact throwing out their men in order to become eligible for the allowance, of preventing men legally recognizing their children and even of conceiving babies for the sole purpose of benefiting from the allowance' (Dagenais 1993: 102). However, these apparently similar reactions to lone parenthood, elicited by similar policies of state support in the two countries, obscure their very different histories of parenting traditions and household formation, which are associated with differing experiences of economic and social development.

In grappling with commonalities and differences, a number of questions can be raised. Are there several trajectories of family forms and household development in evidence throughout the world or variations on a universal theme? Under what conditions is the lone-parent household likely to emerge or its prevalence to increase? Does an increasing proportion of lone mothers or female-headed households within a country or community signal the breakup of the nuclear family or, on the contrary, the breakup of the extended family? Does it reflect increasing exercise of choice and volition, or the abandonment of women by partners and kin, with extra and unwanted burdens being thrust upon them? Is it a measure of increased autonomy or the substitution of one form of dependence for another, with lone parents being assisted by, but also subjected to the surveillance of, the state? Or does such posing of alternatives itself obscure the situation, with divergent and contradictory processes operating not just between countries, or at different times, but for different women, differentially situated, within the same country?

In exploring diversity of family formation and parenting, this chapter will first consider cross-national variation, with reference to aggregate data for a set of selected countries. Differences in the composition, as well as the proportionate significance, of lone parents (or female-headed households) will be emphasized. Factors of variation apply not just between but also within nations, and, in order to examine their impact more closely, two cases – the UK and Zambia – will then be turned to. In attempting to make sense of diversity overall, reference will be made to patterns of economic development as well as to culture and religion. Consideration will also be given to the role of the state, not just in respect of the policy environment it creates, but also to its ideological orientation. Finally, factors particularly facilitating an increase in the proportion of lone parents or female-headed households will be reviewed.

## CROSS-NATIONAL COMPARISONS

Problems with data are immediately encountered when trying to answer the question of how common single or lone parenting really is. Statistics that bear most closely on the issue of parenting relate variously to marital status of parent(s), residence, and head of household, although recourse to these or some combination of them immediately conflates the notion of family with that of household and of household with that of common residence.[4] Comparisons across time or place also suffer from both yawning gaps in the data and a lack of consensus on definitions of key terms, multiplying the hazards of attempting generalizations or presuming to provide a comprehensive picture.

Acknowledging but not attempting to resolve these issues, Table 4.1 has been constructed to highlight some of the diversity in measures bearing on parenting, family formation and household situation. Cases have been chosen in an attempt to illustrate variation both within and across regions. But because the selection is partly a function of data availability, they should not be seen as exemplars of anything so finely defined as a regional or sub-regional type. Moreover, lack of data has prevented the inclusion of cases from large geographical areas, such as Africa and the Near East, and has left a partial picture for Bangladesh, Argentina and Barbados. More recent comparative data on household heads are not widely available beyond those drawn from census returns of 1980 and 1981 as collated in the special supplement on households and family in the *UN Demographic Yearbook* for 1987.[5] Such figures in any case can only imperfectly yield

*Table 4.1* Measures relating to diversity of parenting for selected countries

| Country | Percentage of all births to women under 20 yrs | Percentage of all brides under 20 yrs | Crude divorce rate, per 1000 pop. | Female heads of house-holds as percen-tage of all heads | Percentage of all house-hold heads who are single fe males |
|---|---|---|---|---|---|
| Argentina | 13.8 (88) | 25.4 (81) | na | 19.2 (80) | 3.9 (80) |
| Barbados | 15.6 (89) | 1.7 (89) | na | 43.9 (80) | 23.5 (80) |
| UK | 7.9 (90) | 7.6 (89) | 3.71 (90) | 25.2 (81) | 5.2 (81) |
| Norway | 4.3 (90) | 3.7 (90) | 2.40 (90) | 37.6 (80) | 8.0 (80) |
| Czechoslov-akia | 13.3 (90) | 32.3 (90) | 2.61 (90) | 22.7 (80) | 3.1 (80) |
| Bangladesh | 11.4 (88) | na | na | 16.8 (81) | 0.2 (81) |
| Singapore | 1.5 (88) | 5.1 (88) | 1.60 (91) | 18.2 (80) | 2.8 (80) |
| Japan | 1.4 (90) | 3.4 (90) | 1.27 (90) | 15.2 (80) | 5.0 (80) |

*Note*: Dates in parentheses
*Source*: Compiled from United Nations (1989, 1992), *Demographic Yearbooks* for 1987 and 1991.

generalizations about lone parenthood given that data on household heads refer only to marital status not to parenthood.[6] Despite these caveats, the data do illustrate the range of variability pertaining to some aspects of marriage, childbearing and household type. Supplemented with information from other sources, they enable certain broad contrasts and comparisons to be drawn.

It is evident from Table 4.1 that there are substantial differences between countries in the age at which marriage occurs and when mothers have their first child. Households headed by females can be found across the board, but their composition as exemplified by the marital status of the head, as well as their relative prevalence, varies considerably. While households headed by single (never-married) women were common in Barbados in the early eighties, for example, in Bangladesh they were exceedingly rare. Such differences are important both for understanding the phenomenon of single parenthood or single household headship and for designing policy responses. A closer examination of some of these cases reveals more of the detail of diversity.

### A Caribbean case – Barbados

There is considerable variability among Caribbean states, with the proportion of all households headed by single females ranging from 1.8 per cent in Cuba to 28.9 per cent in St Vincent and the Grenadines (United Nations 1989). But within the mixture of prevailing forms, one significant strand involves mothers and female kin assuming the most important link within household and family (Olwig 1993: 153). Describing the situation with reference to Monserrat, for example, Pulsipher suggests that:

> The term family means kin connected to you through the female line. Long-term relationships are reserved for maternal consanguineal kin; and males, rather than being disfunctional [sic] in the family or marginalised, as some have suggested, play out their roles most often in their mother/son and sister/brother and uncle relationships.
>
> (Pulsipher 1993: 61)

In Barbados it is common for women to have children early, but for marriage to be delayed, sometimes after several 'child-bearing sexual unions' (Olwig 1993: 153; Besson 1993: 21). Thus the link between procreation, joint parenting and, in some cases, household formation is loose. The houseyard, a typical (though now declining) residential form whose roots are traceable to the domestic space of the slave system, reflects and facilitates this type of parenting. In so far as it still persists, it offers accommodation to the rising educational and career aspirations of young West Indian women, facilitating care of their children by their mothers or other female relatives and thus allowing young women to combine child-bearing with being students and workers, even in the capacity of temporary migrants (Pulsipher 1993: 61).

## South Asia – Bangladesh, Pakistan and India

As illustrated in Table 4.1, the case of Bangladesh contrasts markedly with that of Barbados. In the former, childbirth comes relatively early and almost exclusively within the confines of marriage, which occurs early for women[7] and, according to Duza (1989: 127, 140), is virtually universal, with unmarried women generally being considered redundant. Of females aged 20 to 24 in 1981, only 5.1 per cent remained 'never married'. While almost 17 per cent of households in Bangladesh were female headed in 1981, over half of these heads were widows; only 1.4 per cent were single women (and probably fewer still were never-married lone parents). In Pakistan, female headship was even less common, applying to only 4.3 per cent of households in 1981 (United Nations 1989: Table 35). As in Bangladesh, there was only a minuscule proportion of households (less than 0.5 per cent) headed by single women.

Bharat's analysis of 1981 census data in India found lone mothers to be similarly rare: 4.8 per cent of the female population aged 15 to 49 years and 6 per cent of the ever-married female population. The overwhelming majority of lone mothers – 85 per cent – were widows. No figures are given for unmarried mothers, underlining their paucity – or at least invisibility (Bharat 1986: 57). Across much of south Asia, where lone parenthood has occurred, for whatever reason, the parent has characteristically been absorbed into the extended family. But there are portents of change. Alam (1985) argues that the rise in female-headed households in Bangladesh in the 1980s is largely a reflection of the increasing 'social abandonment of women', partly through a loosening of kinship obligations, ironically through what she refers to as the modernization of patriarchal attitudes toward women, aggravated by a pattern of economic change leading to increased inequality in the agrarian sector and a lack of alternative wage employment.

## East and Southeast Asia – Japan and Singapore

A different pattern from either Barbados or Bangladesh appears to apply, at least at the aggregate level, in both Japan and Singapore, where very few women under the age of 20 years either enter into marriage or have children. In many cases in East and Southeast Asia recent decades have seen progressive and rather substantial rises in age at marriage, with figures for first marriage of females in Peninsular Malaysia, for example, increasing from 19.4 years in 1957 to 22.3 years in 1970 and to 23.8 years in 1980 (Arshat and Mohd 1989: 101). In Singapore the increase was even steeper, from 20.3 years in 1957 to 26.2 years in 1980 and 27 years in 1990 (United Nations 1994: 333).

Households headed by single women are relatively uncommon in both Japan and Singapore. Japan, indeed, has been characterized as having a direction of change in family patterns at odds with that of other industrialized nations, with a declining rate of divorce and a decrease in the proportion of out-of-wedlock births, coinciding with a rise of the nuclear family (Burns and Scott 1994: 32, 110). The proportion of all households headed by females, moreover, declined between 1980 and 1990 (United Nations 1989: 1160–1, 1993: 97–8). Because marriages are less prone to dissolution through divorce in both Japan and Singapore than in many European countries, there is a much larger proportion of female heads who are widows than those who are divorced or separated (United Nations 1989: 1160–2).

## Variation across Europe

Within Europe there are many diverse patterns of marriage, parenting and household formation, as suggested by the cases of Norway, the former Czechoslovakia and the UK – though none of these is necessarily representative of a distinct 'type'. Czechoslovakia, along with a number of other eastern European countries is characterized by earlier child-bearing than elsewhere in Europe but also, and more strikingly, by earlier marriage. In Czechoslovakia 32.2 per cent of brides are under 20 years old, while respective figures for Bulgaria, Hungary, Poland and Romania are 38 per cent, 27.5 per cent, 22 per cent and 29.8 per cent.[8] Though almost a quarter of households in

Czechoslovakia are headed by females, 59 per cent of these are widows, a higher proportion than in Japan or Singapore (United Nations 1989: 1160). Argentinean data in Table 4.1 are remarkably similar to those of Czechoslovakia, save for the fact that there is a greater proportion of brides under 20 years old in the Eastern European case than the South American one.

In contrast, Norway, broadly in common with other Scandinavian countries, is characterized by later marriage and childbirth, though delay in birth of first child is shorter than in either Japan or Singapore. Particularly striking is the high proportion of all households in Norway that have female heads (37.6 per cent), a fifth of whom were single women. The proportion of all households headed by single women in Norway (8 per cent) is, however, considerably smaller than that in some Caribbean islands, suggesting a difference in histories of households and family formation between the two.[9]

Figures for the UK rest between some of the 'extremes' applying in other regions or countries and certainly in respect of the cases of Norway and Czechoslovakia (except as regards divorce). Haskey's (1994) recent analysis of 1991 and 1971 census data, which disaggregates the broad category of lone parent on the basis of marital status, provides an indication of changing patterns and the complexity of changing needs.[10]

The steepest rise in family type was that headed by single lone mothers, which included 1.2 per cent of all families with dependent children in 1971 and 6.6 per cent twenty years later. But almost two-thirds of lone mothers in 1991 were formerly married, with about 36 per cent of lone mothers divorced, 22 per cent separated and 5 per cent widowed. The steepest decline across the twenty-year period was among widows, who had comprised 25 per cent of lone mothers in 1971 (Haskey 1994: 7).

This is a pattern in marked contrast to Barbados, where most lone parents are single, and to India, where most are widows. If there is a signal of 'weakening social fabric' to be detected from the UK statistics, it is not by virtue of abandonment of marriage or a severing of the link between marriage and child-bearing but rather a greater tendency for a breakage of unions through divorce or separation, which may in practice lead to a less permanent status as lone parent than is the case for widows (or was indeed for widows in the UK in former decades). The social fabric appears to be changing shape rather than weakening.

## VARIATION WITHIN COUNTRIES

Alongside those differences in marital status that describe the way in which people become lone parents, there are also other dimensions of variation within countries. Some of these will be explored through reference to the cases of the UK and Zambia. As well as representing countries at different levels of development, these two also illustrate different dominant factors of internal variation: ethnicity in the UK and rural–urban variation in Zambia.

### Different patterns for different ethnic communities in the UK

Data reviewed by Haskey on the prevalence of lone-parent families by geographical area within the UK suggest that higher rates apply in urban than in rural areas, with an indicative contrast of 36.7 per cent in inner London, 19.2 per cent in outer London and 12.4 per cent in Surrey (Haskey 1994: 13). The differences may be partly accounted for by the factor of class, though the picture in respect of this variable is both complicated and difficult to document. There may be a higher propensity for those from poorer families to enter into the category of unmarried parent (at least in the younger age ranges), but entering the status of lone parent – through divorce, separation or widowhood – may also lead to a substantial decline in previous income. Ethnicity is another dimension of diversity. Substantially different patterns characterize black, Asian and white communities – partially but only imperfectly reflecting contrasting aggregate patterns as between the Caribbean, South Asia and Europe.

Recent analysis by Heath and Dale (1994) uses microdata from the 1991 census to detail such differences as they relate to women in the age range 16–35. Lone mothers living outside the parental home were much more common among black than among white women and strikingly rare among Asian women. In the age category 25–29 years, 28.4 per cent of black women were in separate, lone-parent house-holds as against 9.8 per cent of white women and 2.1 per cent of Asian women. In the age band 30–35 almost a third (32.2 per cent) of black women were lone parents living in their own accommodation.

Marriage is a norm strongly adhered to within Asian communities, as is the confining of procreation to the marital union, although their hold on second-generation Asian women shows some signs of loosening. There are some Asian lone mothers living within the parental home, but they are very few: 0.5 per cent of Asian females in the age range 16–20 years and one per cent for the age range 30–35. Rates of cohabitation, with or without children, are also low.

For black women in the UK, it is marriage that is relatively uncommon, at least among those aged between 16 and 35 years. While more black than Asian women cohabit, less than a third of black women aged 25 to 29 in 1991 were *either* married or cohabiting, though this combined figure increased to 43.9 per cent for the age category 30–35. There is also a very loose relationship of motherhood with either marriage or cohabitation among black women. Two-thirds of black mothers aged 16–19 years and 53 per cent of those aged 26–27 years were in lone-parent households. Even in the age range 30–35, lone mothers in separate accommodation were more common than married mothers in conjugal households.

The pattern for young white women in the UK falls between those described by the experience of Asian and black women. However, there is a higher rate of cohabitation among white women than among either one of the other two groups: 16.9 per cent of white women aged 21–24 cohabited in 1991 as against 7.3 per cent of black women and 1.3 per cent of Asian women (Heath and Dale 1994).

## Zambia – the rural–urban divide

Ethnicity is probably of lesser importance in explaining variable patterns of lone parenthood in Zambia than in the UK, though some variation is associated with diverse matrilineal or patrilineal traditions characterizing various tribal and ethnic groups. A more important dimension of internal differentiation in parenting and household formation is the rural–urban divide, in consequence both of the loosening of cultural prescriptions that has accompanied urbanization and of the impact on families of patterns of rural–urban migration.

Public concern in Zambia is less focused on the adequacy of parenting by single mothers than on the economic viability of female-headed households, and it is in terms of household type rather than mode of parenting that data are typically collected. Figures for the number of female-headed households in the country as a whole vary considerably from one source to another, indicative of methodological problems inherent in their collection and resulting in part from the difficulty of defining or demarcating 'household'. There may also be slippage in recording all cases of *de facto* as well as *de jure* household heads. Whereas the *de facto* label may apply to some polygamous households, it increasingly and more importantly applies to situations where a wife has been left to manage – temporarily or on a long-term basis – when her husband migrates to urban areas in search of employment. Some of these cases go uncounted, by appearing to be subsumed within extended kin networks, even though the primary responsibility for household subsistence may rest with the woman. Cases of widows being ostensibly embedded in extended households may also go uncounted, as may those of young unmarried mothers.

In spite of inconsistencies among various sources, there is general agreement that the proportion of households with female heads is smaller in urban areas than in rural areas, 15 per cent as against 23 per cent according to the World Bank sponsored Priority Survey of 1991 (Government of the Republic of Zambia 1993: 40). The breakdown of female heads by marital status also differs as between the hinterland and the towns, with lone female parents or household heads in urban areas more likely to be divorced or separated women,[11] while those in rural areas are more likely to be widowed (Mwila 1981: 6). It follows that lone mothers in towns are likely to be younger than those in rural areas. Female-headed households are among the poorest within the country. The Priority Survey of 1991, covering 10,000 Zambian households, found 70 per cent of female-headed households falling into the category of extremely poor as against 57 per cent of male-headed households – the proportions in both cases are alarming and testimony to the severity of economic hardship weathered by the country throughout the last two decades (Government of the Republic of Zambia 1993). A series of small studies in Northern Province found female-headed rural households typically cultivating smaller parcels of land than those of male heads and suffering from labour and other resource constraints (Geisler *et al.* 1985: 130–1).

Though female-headed households in urban areas are also poor, their situation on average is probably less bleak than that of female heads in rural areas. Migratory patterns leave women in the hinterland particularly exposed to hardship, while traditional forms of kinship regulation have less force in the towns. This means that, when choice enters into patterns of parenting, it is more likely to be exercised within the urban setting by more highly educated women with independent access to income.

Some low-income female-headed households fall within the most vulnerable category, but so too do any multi-couple extended households. Indeed, it is the latter that have experienced the greatest increase in recent years, with the severity of economic conditions exerting pressure on households to absorb additional unemployed adults as well as single siblings and grandchildren (Moser 1994: 91), and this counters the easy assumption that the predominant trend in countries such as Zambia is toward conjugal arrangements and the nuclear family.

There is increasing recognition in Zambia, as elsewhere, that effective policy must be informed by the heterogeneity of female household heads or lone mothers (Geisler 1985: 7). The situation of the widow with young children, subjected to the much maligned but still common custom of property grabbing, or of the wife abandoned by her migrant husband in the rural areas, may be very different from the graduate in the urban area with a secure and well-paid job. Yet in Zambia, as in many other developing countries, the stark reality is of precious little assistance from public sources for any female household heads, whatever their specific circumstances.

## MAKING SENSE OF DIVERSITY WITHIN AND ACROSS NATIONS

An increasing prevalence of the nuclear family has been tied to processes of industrialization, urbanization, westernization and capitalist development (Goode 1963) and the apparent decline of the nuclear family to post-industrial processes. But in some situations, such as migrant labour regimes in southern Africa, or the conditions imposed by contemporary structural adjustment prescriptions, capitalist development simultaneously fosters the nuclear family and creates the conditions for its dissolution. This highlights a complex picture relating to the differences in historical experience that underlie aggregate cross-national variation, as well as differences among communities or between individuals within a country.

Economic change affects household arrangements and patterns of family formation in both facilitating and inhibiting ways and is in turn mediated by other factors. Among them are the encoded beliefs and practice bearing on the family, sexuality, procreation, etc., embodied in 'culture', 'tradition' or indeed 'religion'. As both the product and precursor of change in household arrangements, their articulation with changing economic forms and relations yields many specific variations. The role of the political ideologies in respect of this articulation is often of crucial importance. While referring specifically to Malaysia, Stivens's comment that 'kinship and family have their own history, the effects of a continuous social process of construction through state legislation, economic changes, political action, and the rise of social practices like welfare and public health measures, and class action' (Stivens 1987: 91) has much wider application. Other writers have similarly confirmed the interplay between culture, economy and the state in reference to household and family, while also highlighting the specific role of agency in promoting change or resisting its imposition.

Stacey (1983: 266), for example, refers to the way in which socialism, as a political ideology and economic system, both transformed a traditional patriarchal social order of China and was in turn structured by it. Bozzoli's (1983) discussion of the variable impact of capitalism on gender relations in southern Africa utilizes the phrase 'patchwork quilt of patriarchies' to describe how the effects of colonial capitalism and the domestic struggles waged within it resulted in 'a system in which forms of patriarchy are sustained, modified and even entrenched in a variety of ways depending on the internal character of the system in the first instance'. Besson describes how a 'new conjugal complex' was constructed in the Caribbean in resistance to the system of slavery that destroyed African marital traditions (Besson 1993: 21). Each of these reflects an appreciation of the ways in which ideologies, legal forms and economic processes articulate with existing structures and processes in a complex fashion, involving resistances, stumbles and readjustments. The outcome in any given case cannot be read off from the tenets of an ideology or the assumed requirements of a particular economic system, but is mediated by circumstance and historical experience.

## The impact of religion

Yet ideologies – whether religious or political – may be powerful tools for changing or preserving family and household forms. (Mary McIntosh, Chapter 8 in this volume, analyses this in relation to the UK.) Afshar (1987), for example, notes how the Iranian state referenced Islamic values when introducing new legislation governing marriage and the family following the 1978 revolution, designed to counter what was regarded as the western orientation of the previous regime, and specifically its legislative reforms. The legal age of marriage for females was reduced from 18 years to 13 years. Polygamy was reintroduced and former divorce and custody provisions were overturned, with men being given the virtually exclusive right to divorce at will. Afshar (1987: 75–6) argues that the new regime appropriated marriage and defined it as central to a revolutionary, Islamic morality. Marriage was depicted as not just desirable but essential for young women, with the unmarried at one point being equated with terrorists.

In other cases where Islam is less politicized or the state more secularized, or where social forces are differently arranged, the impact of Islamic law and conventions may take a different form. But Islam, as well as other religions, may still exert a strong influence on norms of family and household formation.

## Socialist agendas and family reform

In charting the transformation of patriarchal forms in twentieth-century China, Stacey (1983: 181, 254) describes a close connection between political agendas and family and household forms in a rather different context. Unlike in Iran, it was not western reforms that were under attack but feudal practices as embodied in Confucian patriarchy. While claiming that China's family policy was essentially developed 'behind the back of its revolutionary theory', she nevertheless describes its success as a consequence of political acumen whereby the previous system was not simply denounced but new or modified forms introduced through a complex process of accommodating, exploiting and then reforming the traditional values of the peasantry. China's socialist revolution, argues Stacey (1983: 258), accelerated some pre-revolutionary processes of family change, but also decelerated or reversed others.

Family reform was recognized as crucial to the socialist agenda in China and was self-consciously oriented towards eliminating the feudal system and introducing, supporting and indeed enforcing a new 'democratic family' system for the ultimate end of stimulating the productive forces (Stacey 1983: 176). The marriage law identified the family as the basic unit of socialist development, and a new family morality was stipulated as the means by which it should operate (Stacey 1983: 187, 230).

Molyneux (1985) shows how state-sponsored refutation of feudal patriarchal forms similarly occurred in a number of socialist countries, arguing that while ostensibly – or even genuinely – based on concern to ensure greater equity in society, they were directed towards not so much a liberatory project with respect to gender relations as the freeing of women's labour for productive work, while also ensuring that women assumed responsibility for their reproductive role. What was defined as feudal patriarchy was strongly denounced and it was replaced by the nuclear family. Overt oppression in families was eliminated but complementary gendered roles prevailed. In such cases the state defined, attempted to codify and frequently policed a form of family and parenting deemed ideologically acceptable, but also consistent with needs of economic development.

## Slave regimes and the colonial state

Stacey (1983) offers the hypothesis that modernization under the auspices of revolutionary socialism may have been less destructive of pre-modern family ties than that under capitalist modernizing processes. As an adjunct to modernization elsewhere – though not itself warranting the label of 'modern' – the slave system was particularly destructive in rupturing pre-existing marital, family and household forms. Procreation in some cases was reduced to the production of human commodities for sale, with mothering becoming an often temporary exercise and fathering regarded as expendable. Marriage, kinship and family forms were reconstructed from within this legacy, not just of disintegration but of calculated obliteration of the integrity of former traditions.

The role of the colonial state as a modernizing force – or the overseer of economic change – also imparted a destructive impact on pre-modern family forms, if perhaps in general less extreme than under regimes of slavery. While in some cases upholding customary law and practice, not least in areas bearing on the family, colonial administrations also invariably imported civil codes from the metropolis, which were in turn frequently supported by the religious ideologies promulgated by missionaries. But their sponsorship or tolerance of particular forms of economic practice – including forced labour and long-distance migrant labour – also had implications for family structures. By removing young adult males from the hinterland, while simultaneously concentrating purchasing power within the new monetary economy in their hands, systems of migrant labour had the capacity both to undermine the authority structures on which the rural extended family were based and compromise the sustainability of any residual nuclear households.

In many cases, a clear preference for the nuclear, monogamous family may have been expressed through the imposition of imported legislation and the gender ideologies adhered to by colonial administrators. Yet the mixture of contradictory forces impinging on families was often played out very much behind the backs of the colonists. There was seldom a deliberate and calculated effort to undermine the 'traditional' family in colonial situations of a degree paralleling that under slavery or indeed under socialist regimes; nor, as Stacey (1983) claims to have been the case in China, was a stable family form typically put in its place. And while old forms were certainly undermined – sometimes in dramatic ways – the articulation between old and imported forms registered some elements of continuity.

Themes of dissolution, conservation, and reconstruction of family forms applied differently among different groups, depending on the manner in which their particular economic experience of colonialism interacted with previously existing cultural and economic forms. But the prevalence of female-headed households, particularly in rural areas, is a dominant feature across many formerly colonized countries. Estimates of the proportion of rural households headed by women range as high as 60 per cent in Mozambique, with figures of 55 per cent for Ethiopia and the Maldives and 50 per cent in the Congo and Angola (Jazairy et al. 1992: 273, 406–7).[12]

The role of the state in enforcing the fracturing of families that such figures reveal was particularly acute in South Africa, where the regulation of movement by pass laws and the creation of homelands, disproportionately populated by the young, the old and females of all ages, were crucial elements of the apartheid strategy. But if women were frequently 'left behind' by their migrant menfolk, they did not merely 'wait' passively (Berger 1992). Many responded to their situation by ensuring economic self-sufficiency for themselves and their children, through their own migration to towns, where they sometimes entered into informal unions, or by obtaining work in the factories that became established in the 'homelands'. For Berger the situation was one of families not simply breaking down but being refashioned in accord with circumstances, with the result bearing some parallels to patterns of kinship and family formation in the Caribbean:

[F]amily relationships were being reconstructed in new ways that stressed the connection among women, children, and other female kin. This reorganisation of family life occurred because so many women became actual or de facto household heads at an early stage of their lives.

(Berger 1992: 244–5)

In commenting on this pattern of 'woman-centred households', Preston-Whyte (1993: 66–7) suggests that for many a fundamental break has occurred between institutions of childbirth and marriage. While marriage is not necessarily shunned, life without marriage constitutes an alternative route through life, albeit one in which children continue to feature prominently.

In this case, as with colonial and post-colonial states more generally, a mixture of patterns is evident, with different trajectories of change operating simultaneously. If the extended family is in some cases being undermined, so too is the nuclear family – existing in truncated form and sustained by often overburdened *de facto* female heads. Moreover, it may be the extended family that is experiencing the greatest rate of increase in recent years, as attempts are made to survive amid shortages of housing, employment and income in the context of structural adjustment. At the least, as Lauras-Lecoh (1990: 489) observes in her overview of family trends in Africa, enlarged families, 'midway between the extended family of blood relations and small family units', are holding their ground. And while the prevalence of female-headed households and of lone motherhood is sometimes taken as a measure of deprivation, it may also be an expression – at least in some cases – of the crafting of survival strategies based on reciprocity and assistance among female kin.

## FACTORS FACILITATING THE RISE OF FEMALE-HEADED HOUSEHOLDS

In seeking to isolate the conditions that facilitate the rise of female-headed households across time and place, which may also bear on the variable prevalence of lone mothering, Momsen (1991: 26) has pointed to forms of inheritance, control of property and economic opportunities. Female-headed households, she suggests, are more likely to emerge where property is individual rather than corporate and where women are able to own and control property and have independent access to subsistence opportunities through work, inheritance or state provision. She notes, moreover, that subsistence opportunities must be reconcilable with child care – an important qualification in respect of female heads who are also mothers – and adds that the income realizable through subsistence activities must not be markedly lower than that of men of the same class (Momsen 1991: 26).

In general, then, differing prevalence of female-headed households – or of lone mothers – in different countries, communities or class categories may result from the extent to which an environment enabling their proliferation exists. A facilitating legal framework, a tolerance for diversity in family forms, supportive welfare provision or the possibility of gaining sufficient income through employment to maintain a household and cover child-care costs are all important factors.

Such a formulation, however, applies most fully to lone mother-hood or female headship being entered into by choice. But women find themselves as lone parents or household heads both by their own volition and by default. And even where chosen, such status may not be the choice of first preference, but the best in the context of a mixture of circumstances, among them whether the state provides any support or assistance with housing, child care or general subsistence and the availability of contraception or abortion. The degree of or possibility for choice varies across time, place and community. Preston-Whyte (1993: 69) argues that in contrast to industrialized countries, where some women are choosing to rear their children outside of marriage, many of the lone African female parents in Durban have no choice, but are simply seeking strategies to confront poverty and difficult socio-political circumstances. Many female household heads in the rural areas of developing countries have been thrust into a situation not of their choosing through the desertion or temporary absence of their husbands. In the Caribbean – and elsewhere – where a general tolerance of variable family situations maintains and motherhood continues to carry considerable independent prestige, marriage may remain the dominant ideal (Preston-Whyte 1993: 68) and lone mothers can still be subject to rebuke for their immature and compulsive behaviour (Dagenais 1993: 99). Moreover, the ability to choose for any particular form of parenting or household may be circumscribed by class position Dagenais (1993: 99) comments, for example, that the highest rates of fertility and the highest proportions of women raising their children alone in the Caribbean tend to be among those women least educated and most economically deprived. This indicates not so much choice as a limited scope of alternatives, sometimes entailing dependence on the state as a means of avoiding dependence on individual men. But even in dire circumstances with minimal external forms of support, there is evidence in some cases that if women are not rejecting marriage they are questioning its value, opting to postpone it or choosing to exit from it. Wright's study of women in Lesotho indicated a clear strand of opinion in favour of staying single, associated with complaints that husbands were often inadequate providers, drank too much and beat their wives, and reinforced by the conviction that marriage was not a prerequisite for having children (Wright 1993: 249, 250). In this sense, lone parent-hood may carry different values for those in different social locations, confronting different circumstances, and may be variously seen in a positive or negative light.

## CONCLUSION

The spectre of lone parenthood is often difficult to confront because it conflates so many issues, the significance of which may vary for different groups in different social settings. Anxiety about children born out of wedlock or to very young mothers, problems of lone-household heads being able to provide economic support for their offspring and concern about individuals side-stepping responsibilities and making undue or undeserved claims on the state are among them. It is evident that concern is not always even articulated in terms of lone parenting. Where there is a tendency to equate parenting with mothering, it is not the ability of lone mothers to perform that is questioned but their capacity, given the limited resources they command (see Moore, Chapter 3 in this volume), hence the concern about female-headed households being located among the vulnerable groups in indebted, developing countries. In richer countries, in which welfare structures have been created, it has also been shown that policies themselves encourage forms of parenting deemed inappropri-ate or unacceptable (see Millar, Chapter 5 in this volume, and Edwards and Duncan, Chapter 6).

This review of diversity across and within nations in the nature of parenting and household formation has pointed to the complexity of patterns and the need to see any given case – or community within it – in the context of historical experience, itself influenced by differing circumstances of state and economy and mediated by differing political and religious ideologies. The complex picture that results exhibits some commonalities but also many contradictory tendencies. No policy response can be effective that ignores its varied dimensions.

## NOTES

1   Members of the Organization for Economic Cooperation and Develop-
    ment (OECD) are Australia, Austria, Belgium, Canada, Denmark,
    Finland, France, Germany, Ireland, Italy, Japan, New Zealand, the
    Netherlands, Norway, Sweden, Switzerland, the United Kingdom and
    the United States.
2   Increases in the proportion of families headed by lone parents have
    characterized many countries in recent years, though rates of change
    have varied considerably. The greatest increases have been in the former
    USSR (with the figure doubling from about 10 per cent in the early 1970s
    to about 20 per cent by the mid-1980s) and the USA (where the figure
    stood at about 24 per cent in the mid-1980s). In Sweden, which had the
    highest figure in the industrialized world in the early 1970s (15 per cent),
    the increase to 17 per cent by the mid-1980s was much less pronounced.
    Much lower proportions, accompanied by only minimal increases,
    characterized France, where the figure was 10 per cent in the mid-
    1980s, and Japan, where it hovered around 4 per cent throughout the
    1980s (Burns and Scott 1994: xii–xiii).
3   In fact, only a minority of cases fit the stereotype of miscreant char-
    acteristically invoked by the critics – of young, unmarried mothers. Less
    than 4 per cent of all lone mothers in the UK were under the age of 20 in
    1991 (Haskey 1994: 10).
4   There is a considerable literature on the lack of coincidence between
    household and family and on the limitation of available statistics for
    revealing the complexities of household formation. See Lauras-Lecoh
    (1990) for a general discussion of the situation in Africa, and the *UN
    Demographic Yearbook 1987* for a lengthy account of varying definitions
    of household and head of household across nations. For specific discus-
    sion of female-headed households in developing countries, see Youssef
    and Hetler (1983).
5   The UN's Special Issue of the *Demographic Yearbook on Population,
    Ageing and the Situation of Elderly Persons*, published in 1993, gives more
    recent data on female-headed households, though for only eight coun-
    tries. In view of the small number of cases and the fact that no breakdown
    of female heads by marital status is provided, I have relied on material
    included in the 1987 volume. If now somewhat dated, it remains the most
    comprehensive set available and serves the purpose of indicating the
    range of variability across nations, which is the primary concern of this
    chapter.
6   While disaggregating the category of lone parenthood in respect of
    marital status is crucial for a full appreciation of the nature and
    variability of the needs of those included within it, finding statistics that
    permit such disaggregation and particularly allow for cross-national
    comparisons in this area is fraught with difficulties. Most statistics are
    organized around legal status – unmarried, married, divorced, sepa-
    rated, widowed – with some of these sometimes merged. Other forms of
    union – variously described as consensual, cohabitation, common-law or

'traditional' marriage – which may well involve joint parenting, are not always included. And when utilized, terms vary from one case to another.

7   In terms of international comparisons, the average age of marriage for females in Bangladesh, at 16.7 years in 1980, was particularly low (United Nations 1994: 328).

8   Calculated from United Nations 1992: Table 24.

9   In some Scandinavian countries, marriage is far from universal; consensual unions are increasingly regarded as a legitimate option for couples and a considerable proportion of all births can be classified as out-of-wedlock. At the same time, teenage pregnancies are very rare. See Burns and Scott (1994) for a detailed analysis of patterns of mother-headed families in Sweden.

10   The composition of lone mothers by marital status differs substantially between countries. While in general the proportions who are unmarried and divorced or separated have increased and the proportions of those who are widows have declined, the amount of change varies. In Sweden, with perhaps the highest figure among industrialized nations, the proportion of lone mothers who were unmarried increased only slightly from about 35 per cent in 1970 to about 39 per cent in 1980. In France the respective figures over this period were about 12 per cent and 18 per cent. And while only about 5 per cent of lone mothers were widows in Sweden in 1980, the figure in France remained high at about 30 per cent, albeit declining from about 45 per cent in 1970 (Burns and Scott 1994: 6).

11   Eighty per cent of female heads in Moser's Kamwala sample were divorced or separated (Moser 1994: 27).

12   Though not specified, these figures are presumably calculated on a combined *de facto/de jure* basis.

# Chapter 5

# Mothers, workers, wives
## Comparing policy approaches to supporting lone mothers

*Jane Millar*

It has been just over twenty years since the Finer report on lone-parent families in the UK was published (Finer 1974). The report was the first attempt to consider in detail the policy implications of changing family structure and remains the most detailed and comprehensive account of the circumstances of lone parents. However, it had only a very limited impact on policy. Few of the recommendations were put into practice and the approach adopted by Finer – that the growth in lone parenthood reflected a welcome liberalization of the institution of marriage and that the most pressing issue was the poverty experienced by lone mothers and their children – seems very far indeed from the official view today. In fact, for most of the twenty years following the Finer report, policy towards lone parents has changed very little. The most tangible change has been the targeting of some additional help towards these families within existing benefit provisions: one-parent benefit as a small supplement to child benefit, less stringent means tests for family income supplement (later family credit) and housing benefit, more recently the lone parent premium in the income support scheme (Millar 1994a).

But following this long period when policy has been relatively static, the early 1990s have seen some significant changes, which, if successful, will create a very different structure of support for lone-parent families in the future. Central to the thinking that provided the framework for these policy changes was the argument that lone parenthood was imposing an unacceptably high cost on society as a whole, both directly and indirectly. The direct costs include the rising social security bill for lone parents, which tripled in real terms during the 1980s, as the proportion of lone mothers receiving supplementary benefit or income support rose from about half to over three-quarters, while the proportion of lone parents employed fell to below four in ten, and the proportion receiving maintenance from their former partners fell from about one half to just under a quarter. Lone-parent families also made up an increasing proportion of homeless families and families living in the otherwise dwindling public housing sector.

The indirect costs are not so readily quantifiable but they supposedly arise from the status of lone parenthood itself. As analysed in more detail in other chapters here (particularly Burghes, Chapter 9, Phoenix, Chapter 10, and Roseneil and Mann, Chapter 11), lone parents, especially single mothers, are seen by some as the epitome of the failure of the family: irresponsible mothers whose motives – and capability – for motherhood are questionable and who 'choose' a life of benefit-dependency. These women are 'wedded to welfare' for both their incomes and their homes. Their 'selfish' choices mean that their children grow up damaged by the lack of a father and this has a negative impact throughout society as a whole (Dennis and Erdos 1992; Morgan 1995). These fathers too have come in for an increasing share of condemnation, for refusing to accept their responsibilities to their children and happily leaving the taxpayer to meet the costs of their personal choices: costs that include rising rates of juvenile delinquency and crime, drug abuse and second-generation unemployment and lone parenthood. Here is the dependency culture indeed.

Thus the key policy objective has become to reduce the costs of lone parents both in the short term (by reducing dependency on income support) and in the longer term (by making separation more costly and hence perhaps marriage more attractive). The key legislation was, of course, the 1991 Child Support Act. The provisions of the Act were twofold: first to get more separated fathers to pay higher amounts of child support, and second to get more lone mothers into employment. Thus the aim of the legislation was to change the balance of financial support of lone mothers – to reduce the role of the state in providing that support, to increase the role of fathers through higher child maintenance payments, and to encourage greater self-support through employment.

The relationship between these three potential sources of income – earnings, benefits, maintenance – is central to analysing the nature of the support offered by the welfare state to lone mothers. It thus provides a framework to compare the policies of different countries. Just as the number of lone-mother families has been rising in the UK for the past two decades and more, so other countries have also seen an increase in the number of such families. The UK and Denmark have the highest rates of lone parenthood among the European Union countries, at 15–17 per cent in the late 1980s when the EU average was estimated at about 10 per cent (Roll 1992). Even countries like Ireland – where there was no civil divorce before 1996 – have seen increases in marital separation and unmarried motherhood and so rising proportions of lone mothers (Millar *et al.* 1992; McCashin 1993). Lone mothers make up a significant proportion of all families in the Scandinavian countries and in the English-speaking countries (OECD 1990, 1993). Table 5.1 summarizes these figures.

Widowhood has generally declined as a factor leading to lone motherhood. The most common route into lone parenthood is marital breakdown (divorce and separation), although unmarried motherhood accounts for a rising proportion of the total in some countries, the UK and the USA included. Thus the issue of how to support lone mothers, and especially the 'new' group of non-widowed lone mothers, is an issue for policy in many countries. What role should the state play? What role should the separated parent play? And what role should the lone mother herself play? This chapter seeks to review the policy responses in different countries to these three questions. The objectives are first to describe the nature of the support available to lone mothers in different 'welfare state regimes', and second to examine the ways in which assumptions about gender roles affect welfare provisions.

*Table 5.1* Proportion of all families with children under 18 headed by a lone parent: various countries late 1980s/early 1990s

| European Union countries | (%) |
| --- | --- |
| UK | 17 |
| Denmark | 15 |
| France, Germany | 11–13 |
| Belgium, Ireland, Luxembourg, Netherlands, Portugal | 9–11 |
| Greece, Spain, Italy | 5–6 |

| OECD countries | (%) |
| --- | --- |
| USA | 21 |
| UK, Sweden* | 15 |
| Australia, Austria, Canada, Finland | 13 |
| Netherlands | 11 |

*Note:* * 1985
*Sources*: Roll 1992; OECD 1993

## SOCIAL SECURITY BENEFITS FOR LONE MOTHERS

Most countries recognize the costs of children to some extent in their social security systems (Bradshaw *et al.* 1993; Wennemo 1994), and where universal child benefits or family allowances are provided, lone mothers are entitled to receive these. Eligibility for these benefits is thus on the basis of their status as *mothers* or as carers for children, not specifically because of their status as *lone* mothers. Similarly, where schemes of means-tested child benefits or family allowances exist, these include lone mothers on the basis of their status as *poor families*. Of the fifteen countries included in the study by Bradshaw *et al.* (1993),[1] eleven had a universal family allowance scheme and ten had one or more means-tested schemes for families with working parents. However, although the eligibility of lone mothers to these benefits is through their status as mothers and/or poor families, some countries offer additional payments to lone-parent families. This is true in Denmark, France, Greece, the UK and Norway for universal schemes and in Greece and Australia for means-tested schemes (Bradshaw *et al.* 1993). In addition, the level of support offered to lone parents through these schemes will vary according to the structure of the benefit; for example, schemes that exclude first children (as in France) or pay more for large families (as in the Benelux countries) will pay proportionately less to lone parents, who usually have smaller families than couples.

Designated benefits for lone mothers, where entitlement is specifically related to status as a *lone parent*, are relatively uncommon, except in the case of widows. Widows' benefits and pensions are usually provided as contributory benefits, on the basis of the husbands' contributions, and are intended to replace his earnings. Entitlement to these is, therefore, on the basis of the status of *wife*. Most countries make such provisions, although this is no longer true in Denmark, and the UK restricts these benefits only to widows with children.

There are, however, other examples of benefits specifically for lone parents: Australia, Ireland, Norway and France all provide a 'lone-parent benefit' of some sort. Eligibility relates to the status as *lone parent*, although the structure of these benefits varies quite significantly across the different countries. In Australia all benefits are means-tested but separate benefits are available for different categories of claimant, including lone parents (the 'supporting parent's benefit'). Similarly in Ireland both social insurance and social assistance benefits are divided into separate benefits and lone parents have special entitlements in both schemes (the 'deserted wives benefit', the 'deserted wives allowance' and the 'lone-parent benefit'). In Norway the 'transitional benefit' is paid to lone parents for one year after becoming a lone parent or until the youngest child is aged ten. It is means-tested but does not cease on cohabitation. In France the 'allocation de parent isolé' performs something of a similar role; it is paid for one year after separation if the children are aged over three or until the youngest child reaches the age of three (and for an unmarried mother the benefit would start with the birth of the child and continue for three years).

What these designated lone-parent benefits have in common is that they all allow lone mothers to stay at home and care for their children, up to minimum school-leaving age in Ireland and Australia, up to age ten in Norway, and up to age three in France. They are thus intended as wage replacement benefits, to allow lone mothers to be full-time mothers. It is, of course, not essential that a designated benefit be created to fulfil this objective; in the UK income support is payable to lone parents, without requiring them to be eligible for work, until the youngest child reaches the age of 16. In the Netherlands, lone mothers are also supported at home through the social assistance scheme (Hobson 1994). However the use of designated benefits does make more visible this function of supporting lone mothers as mothers at home.

It is clear that the most common way to support lone mothers is not through designated benefits, but through the provisions that exist for all families with children. For non-employed lone mothers this will usually mean social assistance benefits, for employed lone mothers universal family allowances and in-work means-tested benefits. It would thus be expected that support for lone mothers would be highest in those countries where support for families with children is highest, and lowest where such general support is low. A number of studies suggest that this is indeed the case; for example, Kahn and Kamerman (1983) found this in their study of family support in the late 1970s. Bradshaw *et al.* (1993) also find this. They calculate levels of support for children by taking cash benefits, tax allowances, health, education and housing benefits. They include a variety of different family types at various levels of earnings. Different countries are more or less generous to different types of family (some support large families better than small, or low earners better than higher earners and so on). Table 5.2 reproduces their 'league table', which is the

*Table 5.2* 'Generosity' of child-benefit package: various countries in average rank order (before housing costs)

| Highest level of support | All families | Lone parents |
|---|---|---|
| | Luxembourg | Norway |
| | Norway | France |
| | France | Luxembourg |
| | Belgium | Denmark |
| | Denmark | Belgium |
| *Middle level of support* | *All families* | *Lone parents* |
| | Germany | Australia |
| | UK | UK |
| | Australia | Germany |
| | Netherlands | Netherlands |
| | Portugal | Italy |
| *Lowest level of support* | *All families* | *Lone parents* |
| | Italy | USA |
| | USA | Portugal |
| | Ireland | Ireland |
| | Spain | Greece |
| | Greece | Spain |

*Sources:* Bradshaw *et al.* 1993: Table 9.14

summary measure of support to families. I have grouped the countries into three bands in order to highlight the way in which general support for children and support for lone parents is highly correlated. Those who are most generous to all families are also most generous to lone parents – Luxembourg, Norway, France, Belgium and Denmark. Those least generous to all families are least generous to lone parents – Italy, the USA, Ireland, Spain and Greece. The pattern also holds if employed and non-employed families are considered separately. Thus, what is important for lone mothers is the level of state support offered to all families with children: it is their claims as mothers, not as lone mothers, that are important.

## PRIVATE TRANSFERS: MAINTENANCE AND CHILD SUPPORT

The introduction of child-support legislation in the UK has been one of the most controversial policy developments of recent years and indeed significant changes have been announced in the scheme after only about eighteen months in operation (Department of Social Security 1995). One of the key objectives of the scheme is to reduce discretion in the award of child maintenance. Thus, instead of the courts fixing maintenance in each case individually, the award is made according to a formula, and responsibility for setting, collecting and enforcing awards is the task of an administrative agency. With high levels of separation and divorce this shift to an administrative system can be seen as an attempt to come to grips with family breakdown as a mass phenomenon (Goode 1993; Garfinkel and Wong 1990). In addition, as the name suggests, child-support schemes usually deal only with the issue of support of children. Settlements between spouses (or partners) are not included but, in most of the countries concerned, child support has followed the establishment of 'clean-break' divorce (i.e. where there is no ongoing financial obligation between divorcing partners).[2] Thus child-support schemes seem to continue a process whereby marriage no longer gives rise to long-term financial obligations but parenthood does (Eekelaar 1991; Fox Harding, Chapter 7 in this volume).

Child-support schemes exist in the USA, Australia, Canada and New Zealand as well as the UK. They seem to be a feature of English-speaking countries or, as the Australian committee reviewing the workings of their child-support scheme put it, they reflect an 'Anglo-Saxon' approach to policy in this area (Child Support Evaluation Advisory Group 1992). These schemes do differ quite significantly in their structures, rules and organization, and these differences affect both the way they operate in practice and how they are viewed in different countries. For example, the Australian and the UK schemes have had rather different outcomes (Millar and Whiteford 1993; Millar 1996). However, what binds these child-support schemes together as a distinctive approach is that they involve the state acting to set and enforce family obligations between parents and children.

This Anglo-Saxon model is not the only approach to providing financial support for the children of separated parents. In Europe, and especially Scandinavia, there is a different approach that has been in operation in those countries for some years – the 'Scandinavian' model (Child Support Evaluation Advisory Group 1992).[3] These schemes use maintenance 'advances' or 'guarantees' to ensure that lone parents actually receive child-support payments and then seek to recoup the costs of these from the other parent. Schemes of this type operate in Sweden, Denmark, Finland, Norway, Belgium, Germany and France. As with child support, the ways in which the schemes work – their coverage, eligibility criteria, duration, level of support given and so on – differ from country to country. Some (for example in Sweden and Denmark) have wide applicability while others (for example in France) are restricted to only certain groups of lone parents. The Swedish scheme can be taken as an exemplar of this approach.

The Swedish child maintenance system starts in the courts or, if the parents can agree, with their settlement, which is ratified by the court. The amount of child maintenance awarded is thus fixed according to individual circumstances and bargaining power but the Department of Social Welfare issues guidelines on how to calculate awards. If payments are then defaulted the lone parent can apply for a maintenance advance from the Department of Social Welfare, which the Department pays and seeks to recoup from the absent parent. Unmarried mothers can also apply for a maintenance advance without having to have a court award. The maintenance advance is flat-rate, tax free and paid regardless of the employment and family circumstances of the custodial parent. Use of the scheme seems quite widespread: in 1985 about 68 per cent of lone parents were receiving an advance, as were about 10 per cent of two-parent stepfamilies. In 1990 maintenance advances were paid for about 15 per cent of all children in Sweden (these figures all from Gustafsson and Klevmarken 1994: 104). Of the total amount paid out in 1984 about 32 per cent was recouped from the absent parent, but this total includes cases where there was no requirement for repayment. If these are excluded then the amount recouped rises to about 78 per cent (*Statistical Report of the Nordic Countries* 1987). However, Gustafsson (1990) reports that the proportion of the advance collected from parents relative to the total paid out was falling throughout the 1970s, although the reasons for this are not clear.

This Scandinavian approach is very different from the Anglo-Saxon model in terms of both underlying philosophy and outcomes. The Anglo-Saxon model places the emphasis on the private responsibility of parents for their children. The state plays a secondary, essentially enforcement, role. This reflects a view that stresses private and individual responsibility backed up, but not taken over, by the state. The success of this approach, in terms of generating incomes for lone parents and their children, thus depends very much on two factors: on how effective that enforcement is and on the capacity of absent parents to pay. The Australian experience suggests enforcement can be significantly improved if sufficient resources are put into doing so. However, the American experience, which is of much longer standing and with more powers of enforcement, only produces collection rates typically in the region of 40 to 45 per cent (Child Support Evaluation Advisory Group 1992), so there are likely to be high administrative costs associated with keeping up payment levels. In terms of capacity to pay, both Australian and American research suggest that separated parents can pay more in child support than they have typically done in the past and still achieve an adequate standard of living. Nevertheless, such payments can rarely be more than a contribution to the incomes of lone parents – few men earn enough to support two households fully – and so even if 100 per cent compliance could be achieved this 'private responsibility' model can only achieve so much in relation to providing adequate support for children.

The Scandinavian model, by contrast, places much greater emphasis on collective support for children and the state plays a primary role in guaranteeing that support. Thus the maintenance obligation has become, in effect, a flat-rate benefit for children living with just one parent. The success, in terms of generating income for lone parents and their children, is therefore not dependent on either the willingness or the capacity of the absent parent to pay but on the level of resources that the government is willing to put into it. In addition, whereas the Anglo-Saxon child-support model acts to enforce the financial dependency of individual women upon individual men, the Scandinavian advanced maintenance model breaks this link; the income of the lone mother does not depend on the actions of the separated father.

Approaches to child maintenance thus cannot be separated from the more general approaches to the support of children in different countries and the extent to which this is seen as a collective or as a private responsibility. This point will be addressed again in the final section, but first we need to look at the third potential source of income for lone mothers: their own employment.

## MOTHERS OR WORKERS?

The extent to which lone mothers are economically active varies substantially across countries, ranging from about three in ten in Ireland and the Netherlands up to eight or nine in ten in countries such as Sweden, Finland and the USA (Table 5.3). To what extent do the different policies across countries account for these differences? Do some countries seek to encourage employment among lone mothers while others seek to discourage it?

Two recent studies have examined whether these differences in employment can be explained by differences in the tax and benefit systems, and specifically whether some countries have systems that offer greater financial incentives for lone mothers to work and hence achieve high employment rates. Mitchell (1992), using Luxembourg Income Study data, concludes that there is no clear association between the apparent financial incentives (as measured by replacement rates and marginal tax rates) and the employment rates. Indeed some countries, such as Sweden, have very high replacement rates (i.e. they offer a lot of support to non-employed lone mothers) alongside

*Table 5.3* Employment rates of lone mothers and all mothers: various countries, late 1980s/early 1990s

| Country | Percentage employed | |
|---|---|---|
| | Lone mothers (%) | All mothers (%) |
| Australia | 45 | 58 |
| Belgium | 49 | 53 |
| Denmark | 74 | 80 |
| France | 68 | 59 |
| Germany | 58 | 44 |
| Greece | 54 | 44 |
| Ireland | 25 | 25 |
| Italy | 59 | 41 |
| Luxembourg | 62 | 38 |
| Netherlands | 29 | 34 |
| Norway | 63 | 77 |
| Portugal | 65 | 60 |
| Spain | 48 | 28 |
| UK | 38 | 59 |
| USA | 61 | 63 |

*Source*: Whiteford and Bradshaw (1994) Table 2.

very high employment rates. Whiteford and Bradshaw (1995) base their analysis on model families (as opposed to the survey data used by Mitchell) but draw the same conclusion: that it is impossible to predict employment rates from differences in the tax and benefit systems. Indeed they note: 'Perhaps the most interesting finding is that in a formal sense work disincentives for lone parents exist wherever there are systems of social assistance. Nevertheless behaviour differs substantially' (Whiteford and Bradshaw 1994: 86).

It is necessary to look outside the tax and benefit system, therefore, in order to understand these variations in employment. Demographic characteristics – age, age and number of children, etc. – play some part. However, these demographic characteristics only seem to account for a small part of the variation between countries (Wong *et al.* 1992; Mitchell 1992). Whiteford and Bradshaw (1994) point out that there is some association between the employment rates for lone and married mothers such that, in general, high employment rates for lone mothers are found where there are high employment rates for married mothers and vice versa. A recent OECD study of lone mothers' employment also looks at this point and, having compared different countries on a number of dimensions, concludes that:

[T]he primary explanation for differences between countries in participation by lone mothers lay in factors affecting mothers in general. These factors include the structure of labour markets, relative availability of full-time and part-time jobs, education and training for women, child care and parental leave... measures which encourage participation by women generally and mothers in particular will lead to higher levels of participation by lone mothers.

(OECD 1993: 64)

Thus, it is argued, policy does make a difference to employment rates of lone mothers but not simply, or primarily, through the tax and benefit system but rather through the range of measures – employment rights, services, education and financial support – that influence the ease with which it is possible to combine motherhood and employment, to be in the title of the OECD report 'breadwinners or childrearers'. However, as the OECD report and Whiteford and Bradshaw (1994) both point out, although there is a correlation between the employment rates for lone and married mothers, there are also countries where lone mothers are more likely to be employed than married mothers, sometimes substantially so. For example, as also shown in Table 5.3, this is the case in Spain (48 per cent for lone mothers and 28 per cent for married mothers), Italy (59 per cent and 41 per cent), Greece (54 per cent and 40 per cent) Luxembourg (62 per cent and 38 per cent), and Germany (58 per cent and 44 per cent). So we need also to account for why this should be the case. If we divide the countries into three broad categories, this helps to understand these differences in patterns of paid work.

1   Countries with high employment rates for both lone and married mothers. Employment is supported by a mixture of services (especially child care), employment rights (especially parental leave arrangements, job protection, and effective equal pay policies), and benefits (especially universal family allowances and maintenance guarantees). The Scandinavian countries plus, to a lesser extent, France and Belgium would fit here.

2   Countries with low employment rates for both lone and married mothers or with low employment rates for lone mothers and high rates of part-time working for married mothers. In these countries there is little support for mothers to enter employment, with low levels of child-care provision, minimal employment rights, and low to middling universal benefits. Married mothers who work thus tend to work part-time and fit in their paid work alongside their domestic work. However, because it is not expected that mothers should be employed, non-employed lone mothers are provided with an income out of work, either from social assistance or designated one-parent benefits. In the absence of much support for employment, staying at home is the most viable option for most lone parents. This group is represented by Ireland, the Netherlands, Luxembourg, the UK and Australia.

3   Countries with low employment rates for married mothers but high rates for lone mothers. These are rather like the second group of countries in that support for mothers to be employed is fairly low (low to middling levels of child care, employment rights and benefits). However, in these countries there is also very little support for those without jobs and without rights to unemployment benefits. Lone mothers without employment thus have to rely either on family support or on low, often discretionary, social assistance benefits. Unlike countries in the first group, which pull lone mothers into employment by positive measures of support, in these countries lone mothers are pushed into employment by the lack of any alternative. The countries of southern Europe are

placed here with (to a lesser extent) Germany and Austria. The USA ought to fit here too, although the employment rates for married mothers are higher than might be expected for the group of countries with this pattern.

The three patterns are likely to have rather different outcomes in terms of poverty rates among lone mothers. The first would be predicted to have the lowest rates of poverty, the second to have relatively high rates of poverty but not the greatest depth of poverty, and the third to have high rates of poverty including the most extreme poverty. There seems to be some evidence for this from studies that have compared poverty rates of lone mothers across different countries. For example, Hobson (1994) calculates that poverty rates for lone mothers are lowest in Sweden, followed by the Netherlands, the UK and Germany with the highest rates in the USA. Mitchell (1992), applying regression analysis to data from the Luxembourg Income Study, simulates the effect on poverty and employment rates for lone mothers in Australia if they faced similar circumstances as lone mothers in Sweden and the USA. She concludes that, if Australian lone mothers lived under the Swedish regime, then many more would be employed and poverty rates would fall substantially. If they lived under the USA regime, again many more would be employed but poverty rates would rise substantially. Getting more lone mothers into employment does not always improve their living standards; it can also mean more poverty and insecurity.

## LONE MOTHERS, GENDER AND WELFARE STATE REGIMES

Some common themes emerge from the discussion of the three sources of income presented in previous sections of this chapter. It was argued in the first section that the state support offered to lone mothers is closely related to the state support offered to all families with children. In the second section it was similarly argued that policies towards child maintenance are related to the extent to which the state accepts collective responsibility for children as opposed to enforcing private responsibility. And finally it was suggested that policies to support the employment of mothers in general are also the most important factor in determining the employment rates of lone mothers. In these cases the treatment given to the needs of mothers in general seems central to understanding the position of lone mothers.

Lone mothers are not so much a separate case but a specific example of how women as mothers are treated in policy in different countries.

Another way to express this is to consider how caring work is treated in different welfare states. The need to incorporate care work into comparative analysis has been at the heart of much of the feminist critique of the analysis by Esping-Andersen (1990) of what he termed the 'three worlds of welfare capitalism'. His approach was based primarily on the relationships between the labour market and the state and the extent to which state provisions 'de-commodify', that is, allow workers to have an adequate standard of living outside the labour market. The focus of this analysis is paid work, and it is not clear how unpaid, caring work fits into this, if at all. Thus the experiences and circumstances of women in different welfare state regimes are not systematically included in the analysis. According to Sainsbury (1994: 3), attempts to introduce gender into this type of comparison can be divided into two main approaches: the first is 'to problematize several basic concepts in the mainstream literature by inquiring how they are gendered ... to utilize mainstream theories and conceptions, and where necessary to refashion them, so as to encompass both women and men'. The second approach has been to 'argue that mainstream theories are fundamentally lacking. Because crucial elements are missing, alternative theories and models are required.'

Perhaps the best known of the latter approaches is the typology constructed by Lewis (1992b), in which she sets out a threefold division of countries that relates to the role attached to the 'male breadwinner'. These are:

1  Strong breadwinner states (e.g. the UK, Ireland). A firm dividing line is made between public and private responsibilities, benefits are used to replace male earnings and there is a lack of benefits and services that would help women work outside the home.
2  Modified breadwinner states (e.g. France). Priority is given to horizontal redistribution between those with and without children, so there are high levels of universal child provision, coupled with a recognition of women's claims as both mothers and workers.
3  Weak breadwinner states (e.g. Sweden). Commitment to dual breadwinners with services and benefits to assist parents – male and female, lone and married – to combine child care and employment.

Lone mothers would receive the highest levels of support in either the modified breadwinner approach (where they benefit from the focus on families and positive employment policies) and in the weak bread-winner approach (where they benefit from policies to integrate parents into employment), and this seems to fit with the above discussion. Lone mothers would fare least well in strong breadwinner states but this category seems very large and undifferentiated, and indeed Lewis argues that 'predicting the treatment of lone mothers in strong breadwinner countries is virtually impossible because their situation defies the logic of the system'. Thus lone mothers might either be treated as mothers (benefits to stay at home) or as workers (incentives to enter the labour market).

However, breaking down the strong breadwinner category in a bit more detail could provide a better predictor of the treatment of lone mothers. The analysis above suggests that we need to consider the way in which the earnings of the male breadwinner are replaced, in particular whether this is by means of social insurance or social assistance. Countries with a strong breadwinner/social insurance model replace male earnings with social insurance benefits to cover contingencies such as unemployment, sickness and retirement. Social assistance plays a limited, perhaps discretionary role. The prediction for lone mothers would be relatively high rates of employment for negative rather than positive reasons – the lack of social assistance would give little choice. Germany fits this pattern very well. By contrast a strong breadwinner/poverty relief model replaces male earnings with means-tested benefits intended to meet family needs. The prediction for lone mothers would be low employment rates because social assistance would offer an income, albeit low, for those outside the labour market. The UK and Ireland would fit here. Thus it is important to consider the extent to which benefits are mainly contributory, and hence rest on labour market participation, or are means-tested, and hence rest on demonstrating need.

Focusing specifically on lone mothers, both Cass (1992) and Hobson (1994) also seek to analyse how caring work is recognized in different welfare states. Cass discusses three main models. The 'needs-based welfare state regime' enables women to stay at home and provide care but only in the context of both low wages and low benefits (Norway and Australia). The 'market-centred welfare state' gives caring work little support but at the same time leaves support for paid work to the market (Austria and the USA). The 'liberal welfare state regimes' partially recognize caring work but also leave support for paid work largely to the market (the UK). Similarly, Hobson (1994) contrasts policies in Sweden (a 'parent–citizen–worker' model), where all parents are expected to be in employment and supported in their dual role by the state, with the Netherlands (a 'mother–carer–citizen' model), in which lone mothers are paid a benefit to stay at home and care for their children. These represent two different policy logics in relation to the role of mothers. In Germany, she argues, policy is based on defining women not so much as mothers but as wives: their entitlement is through their husbands and so women without husbands receive very little financial support as full-time carers but nor do they receive support to go into employment. And finally, in the USA, 'work and welfare' are kept very separate, with little support for employment and those on welfare are seen very much as undeserving and dependent.

The relationships between family, state and labour market, where we started this chapter, are clearly very complex in character and not easy to disentangle. Different studies have tended to highlight different aspects, and this to some extent reflects the fact that the studies have looked at various combinations of countries. There is a need for a more systematic analysis across a wider range of countries. The factors that should be examined in more detail are, however, becoming clearer. These include whether claims are on the basis of status as wives, mothers or workers; whether these are established as universal citizenship rights or selective needs-based rights; the extent to which rights are defined in relation to paid employment; the nature of social rights to services as well as individual rights to benefits; the nature of the obligations that family members are deemed to owe to each other and the role that the state plays in either guaranteeing or enforcing these.

Not only do assumptions about gender roles influence the development and nature of social policy but gender relations are also themselves affected by the nature of welfare provisions. Thus the concept of gender can be either 'explanandum or explanans' (Busse-maker and van Kersbergen 1994: 9), both cause and consequence, in our understanding of the nature of welfare states. Child-support legislation, for example, reflects a particular view of the gender roles, with men as financial providers and women as family carers (Lister 1994; Millar 1994b), but at the same time it helps to create a particular relationship of dependency between individual men and women (Clarke *et al.* 1994b; Burgoyne and Millar 1994). Policies that support lone mothers to stay at home and care for their children rather than take up paid employment are a reflection of a particular view of the nature of motherhood, but at the same time they are part of the process that constructs the experience of motherhood through the choices that are, and are not, open to lone women with children. Thus it is also important to consider the ways in which different policy regimes construct the experience of lone motherhood.

Finally, moving away from the theoretical to the policy implications of these comparisons, two points stand out. First, comparing different approaches to the support of lone mothers draws attention to what lone mothers have in common with married mothers rather than what separates them. There are common needs for support if they are to take paid employment, common needs for financial support to help meet the costs of children, even perhaps common needs for mechanisms to give them entitlement to male incomes. Gender rather than family status is the key variable in understanding the situation of lone mothers. Second, almost everywhere lone mothers have a higher than average poverty risk. The main, but still partial, exceptions are countries such as Sweden and Denmark, where gender equality has been a much more central goal of policy. Traditional expectations of gender roles within the family still shape policies in many countries and, while this is the case, lone mothers are likely to remain poor.

## NOTES

1   The fifteen countries were Belgium, Denmark, France, Germany, Greece, Ireland, Italy, Luxembourg, the Netherlands, Portugal, Spain, the UK, Australia, Norway and the USA.
2   One strong area of criticism of the UK scheme has been that it overturns previous 'clean-break' settlements.
3   Using labels such as 'Anglo-Saxon' and 'Scandinavian' points up similarities between countries but can also serve to mask differences. For example, Leira (1992) shows that the Norwegian approach to child-care policy is quite different from that of Denmark and Sweden.

# Chapter 6

# Rational economic man or lone mothers in context?

## The uptake of paid work

*Rosalind Edwards and Simon Duncan*

Lone mothers, caring for dependent children, are a rising proportion of the population in western Europe. Poverty and dependence on state benefits are increasingly important characteristics of lone-mother families in Britain, as compared with most other west European countries. Over 60 per cent now have incomes below half the national average, and almost 70 per cent rely on state benefits for the bulk of their income (Roll 1992).

Although state benefit levels in some west European countries are more generous than in Britain, where benefit levels mean that those who wholly or partially rely on them tend to exist on very low incomes, a major explanation for lone mothers' economic marginalization seems to be their decreasing uptake of paid work.

In 1990, only 39 per cent of lone mothers in Britain were employed, with just 17 per cent in full-time paid work, as compared with around 50 per cent in employment in the mid-1970s, 25 per cent full-time. Over the same period, uptake of part-time and full-time paid work by partnered mothers increased substantially, to outstrip lone mothers' employment rates. These differentials operate independently of the age of children (where more lone mothers now have pre-school-age children).

In all the other west European countries (except for Ireland and the Netherlands), there are much higher rates of employment for lone mothers, especially for full-time work (Roll 1992). Similarly, in the rest of western Europe usually more lone mothers are in paid work than married mothers. Lone mothers in Britain thus appear to exhibit increasingly 'economically irrational' behaviour in comparison with their west European counterparts. This has given rise to a debate in Britain, focused around two main discourses (see also McIntosh,

Chapter 8, Phoenix, Chapter 10, and Roseneil and Mann, Chapter 11, all in this volume, and Edwards and Duncan 1996).

In one discourse, lone mothers are seen as a threat to society, morally as well as financially; they are formative members of an underclass that has willingly removed itself from legitimate economic rationality and mores, turning instead to state benefits, the unofficial economy, and even crime. In the other discourse, lone mothers are seen as a social problem; they want to behave in an economically rational way and take up paid work to better provide for themselves and their children, but the structure and nature of the British welfare state prevent them from doing so.

The first discourse seeks to remove the social threat by penalizing lone mothers, forcing them to act in a legitimate, economically rational way. Reducing benefits, for example, will force them into paid work or dissuade them from having children they cannot support 'out of wedlock' in the first place. In contrast, the second discourse proposes welfare reforms to alleviate the perceived constraints on economically rational behaviour. Thus changes to the benefit system should ensure that lone mothers are better off in paid work than they are living on benefits, and on increased provision of publicly funded child care (to levels commensurate with other European countries) to remove a fundamental block to taking up full-time employment.

The solutions associated with both discourses operate with a simple stimulus–response model of social action. They are based on a 'rational economic man' assumption (usually more explicit in welfare economics and more implicit in social policy analyses). Individual economic agents maximize their personal welfare based on cost–benefit calculations,[1] and national social policy is assumed to be dominant in setting the stage for this. Change the stimulus (such as benefit levels or child-care provision), the economic calculus changes, and lone mothers will respond appropriately (by taking up paid work). Lone mothers' own capacities for action, in relation to a variety of social contexts and settings, are shut out. This point is all the more important because, as Bradshaw and Millar (1991: 33) note, there is actually little coherent empirical knowledge about how and why lone mothers take up employment or do not.

In this chapter, we argue that it is crucial to take account of the fact that the overwhelming majority of lone parents are women who are mothers, and who socially negotiate particular 'gendered moral rationalities' that operate in particular settings and in ways different from individualized economic rationality. Fatherhood is subject to very different moral rationalities, and indeed British lone fathers are far more likely to work full-time and to bring up their children in better material circumstances (Popay and Jones 1990).

National policy *does* provide one context for lone mothers to take up paid work, but social processes do not operate *only* at the level of the nation state. In our analysis of the constraints on and opportunities for lone mothers' employment, we need to envisage a more complex context–action structure.

Social contexts other than national policies include constraining or enabling gendered moral rationalities and identities with different prescriptions about the relationship of motherhood and paid work. These moral rationalities and identities are held and negotiated by different social groups, including lone mothers themselves, and are often located within support networks in particular neighbourhood settings. Similarly, gendered divisions of labour within local labour markets structure both the supply of jobs and social expectations of working for a wage, and provide another influential context for lone mothers' decisions about paid work.

In the following sections we explore each of these contexts, demonstrating the considerable variability in lone mothers' employment by social group and geographical setting, drawing on data from our ongoing research into the processes underlying lone mothers' uptake of paid work.[2] Finally, we examine how state welfare regimes feed into these processes by positioning lone mothers as workers and/or mothers. This gives a complementary angle to the discussion undertaken by Millar in Chapter 5 of this book.

## RATIONAL ECONOMIC DECISION MAKING

The concept of rational economic decision making, and what factors are relevant to and constitute it, are not neutral and gender-free. In particular, 'rational economic man' is a self-contained uncontextualized and emotion-free individual agent, whose actions are governed and calculated by the self-interested drive to maximize economic well-being to himself (and, perhaps, to members of his family). Even where it is acknowledged that economic agents live in households, these are seen as gender-free economic units, who rationally allocate their differentiated labour (to paid work, household work and so on) so as to maximize resources. Social relations within and between households are not seen as important.

In the public, male sphere of the market, the model of individual selfishness is assumed to be the most rational. In contrast, in the private, female sphere of the family, a collective rationality of duty and tenderness is assumed. Not only are these public–private assumptions deeply gendered, they are also inaccurate. The public sphere of markets could not operate without collective social behaviour and mores (Hodgson 1988). Similarly, the incentives for paid work are as much social as economic. In a like manner, the private sphere of family life contains instrumental and individualized interactions over resource use and allocation, as much as it is concerned with intimacy and connection (Ribbens and Edwards 1995). Furthermore, what happens in one sphere interacts with the other, with men and women differentially constituted with respect to various sorts of markets, states and families (rather than there being one version of the market, the family and the state).

The assumption that lone mothers can be regarded as rational economic men is best exemplified in an influential body of work carried out (naturally enough) by econometricians (for example, Dilnot and Duncan 1992; Ermisch and Wright 1991; Jenkins 1992; Walker 1990). The emphasis is on lone mothers as an amalgam or set of individually specific variables (age, qualifications, age of youngest child, entitlement to benefits, receipt of maintenance, housing tenure and so on). Through statistical analysis of large data sets (derived, for example, from the General Household Survey or the Labour Force Survey), the aim is to measure how far, and in what ways, these individual attributes predict lone mothers' propensity to participate in the labour market. It would then be possible to estimate how social policy alterations (for example, changing benefit or maintenance levels) would affect relative participation rates.

One particular problem for these models is the key role, under-pinned by notions of rational economic man, given to the wage commanded by different attributes. It is this wage that is seen to best describe the power of each attribute variable in accounting for participation in the labour market. Most lone mothers, however, do not have paid work, so in the majority of cases it is not possible to correlate wage variation directly with attribute variation when producing statistical equations. Thus analysts have to estimate the wages that non-participating lone mothers would be expected to obtain in relation to their attributes. Different analysts tend to carry out this procedure in different ways, and also do not include the same range of variables (depending on the particular data set drawn upon), so the statistical results vary substantially, and sometimes in contradictory ways, in each account. Thus Ermisch and Wright (1991) emphasize the labour market in explaining lone mothers' declining employment, Walker (1990) emphasizes the benefit structure, and Jenkins (1992) stresses the age of youngest child and childcare costs, plus a range of 'non-economic' (and implicitly inexplicable) factors.

It is not our aim here to comment comprehensively on the explanatory limitations of econometric modelling, some of which may be accepted by econometricians themselves. Rather, we want to take issue with the theoretical assumption used in these models, that lone mothers act as rational economic men, and with the concomitant neglect of social process. Lone mothers are seen as making individual, economically rational calculations about what wage their resources (educational level, previous occupational experience, etc.) will bring them in the labour market, as set against the costs (paying for child care, loss of housing benefit, etc.), and as judged in relation to benefit levels. They then make the decision to take up employment, or not, on the basis of this calculation. Having made this assumption, all that remains, econometrically, is to estimate what effect these variables exert on the employment decision.

The model of rational economic man also underpins much research in the social policy tradition. One example is the influential body of work advocating an expansion of day care to allow lone (and other) mothers to take up paid work (for example, Cohen and Fraser 1991; Holtermann 1992). Here, cost–benefit analyses are employed to estimate the financial results for both state expenditure and lone mothers' incomes. Public money spent on child care is shown to be a good investment for the state, bringing returns in the form of increased revenue from taxation and reduced outlays on lone mothers' income support. Lone (and other) mothers are shown to have an incentive to take up employment because affordable child care means they will be financially better off.[3] The assumptions about lone mothers' employment behaviour are similar to the econometric work, but now the focus is more squarely on national social policy rather than individuals in the labour market. Cohen and Fraser (1991), however, in their calculations, do make allowances for some lone mothers not to make such an economically rational decision. As such, they implicitly acknowledge that other (gendered) forces are also at play, although they do not appear to see these as varying by social group and by social setting.

The model of rational economic man assumes an empowered individual able to act alone and to carry out conscious planning to maximize financial gain in taking up paid work. This is imbued with masculinist, class-based and ethnocentric assumptions. Social factors and various gendered beliefs about the compatibility of motherhood and paid work, which can lead to different conceptions of what is a 'rational choice' (Hollis and Nell 1975), are not seen to play a part. (This is despite the British state itself having long had dilemmas over its stance towards lone mothers – Bradshaw 1989.) So, for example, Jenkins (1992) does not regard black lone mothers' greater propensity to take up paid work as related to their ethnicity (by their socially held conceptions of motherhood in relation to paid work) but as a function of their tendency to have high levels of educational attainment, which in turn places them in a more favourable position in the labour market (in terms of the wage they can receive). That black (mainly African-Caribbean and African) women generally may attain educational qualifications because, as a social group, they are more likely to see motherhood and paid work as integral, and wish to better place themselves in a racially (as well as sexually) discriminatory labour market (as we discuss again below), does not enter into the picture.

In order to understand the process of lone mothers' uptake of paid work, we must move away from a focus on individuals as separate selves (implicitly powerful and economically autonomous males) towards an understanding of gendered institutional and social processes, and the expectations and beliefs shared by social groups that may produce differentiated notions of rational courses of action.

## GENDERED MORAL RATIONALITIES IN CONTEXT

Economic calculations, rather than an asocial economic rationality, are a factor in lone mothers' decision to enter the labour force or live on benefits. They are not, however, the only form of rationality at work, and may be overridden by other ways of making sense of the world. Carling (1991) has discussed the ways in which a rational-choice approach to understanding human action can go beyond merely market-based economics to include independently acting issues around gender. In particular, family life, and especially the combination of motherhood with other roles, is not easily understood on the basis of economic or means–ends rationality (Edwards and Ribbens 1991; Finch 1994).

As pointed out earlier, lone mothers – in common with other women in their social groups and networks – can hold particular understandings about their identity both as mothers and as lone mothers. These understandings about the identity and responsibilities of mothers can be termed 'gendered moral rationalities'. Some of these rationalities may sit comfortably with models of economic rationality; others do so less easily (see Carling 1991). Data from our research into the processes underlying lone mothers' uptake of paid work illustrate these.

Some lone mothers may give primacy to the moral benefit of physically caring for their children themselves over the financial benefits of undertaking paid employment. This moral rationality is socially sustained by norms held in common with others in their social group and local social network. For example, Susan is a white, working-class woman with two children under five, living on a large council estate on the outskirts of Brighton. She says she would 'love' to have paid work as she thinks she would be financially better off, but she has no-one to look after her children. Her own mother, who lives nearby and is very important in Susan's life, is not in employment. Nevertheless, she would not look after Susan's children while Susan worked. Her mother believes that mothers should stay at home and look after their children, as she did, and – like Susan – does not approve of leaving children with 'strangers'. So, even though Susan would respond to a questionnaire by saying she did want paid work, if she did pursue this course of action it would cause tremendous problems in her relationship with her mother, so important in her everyday life. Taking up paid work is seen as morally wrong; even if it is economically rational at an individual level for Susan, it is socially irrational. Here, identities as worker and good mother can be in conflict and are difficult to balance.

In contrast, other lone mothers may see financial provision through employment as one part of their moral responsibilities towards their children. Again this can be sustained socially with others in their social group and networks. For example, Rachel is a Ugandan woman, who also has two children, one of whom is under five, and lives in local authority housing in inner London. She believes that mothers should 'go out to work to earn money and look after the children'. Rachel is currently studying so that she can get a good job in order to 'care adequately' for her children, who attend the college crèche. She gets support and encouragement for her views and actions from her close circle of friends, mainly also African. (The majority of her relations live in Uganda.) For Rachel, a very different gendered moral rationality is in play from the one Susan has to negotiate. It is a moral rationality in which looking after your children encompasses providing for them financially through paid work. Here, identities as worker and good mother are reconciled.

Lone mothers' individual economic calculations thus need to be placed in the framework of gendered moral rationalities that are constructed, negotiated and sustained socially in particular contexts. This is in obvious contrast to dominant economic models of rationality, which see the decision to take up paid work as individually made on the basis of calculations of financial loss and gain.

## NEIGHBOURHOODS AND SOCIAL NETWORKS

There are significant variations between neighbourhoods in lone mothers' rates of employment. For example, Brighton and Hove (two contiguous District Councils) lie near the national average, with 40 per cent of lone mothers in paid work, 14 per cent full-time. Within these areas, though, ward rates (taken as measurement units) varied from 23 per cent to 62 per cent for employment as a whole, and 6 per cent and 25 per cent for full-time work (based on 1991 Census data). Such spatial differences partly overlap with, and reflect, the social groups of lone mothers in an area. Thus it is important to examine the features of the neighbourhood-based contexts that may facilitate or constrain lone mothers' employment.

The local setting can be a particularly important and relevant part of mothers' lives – a socially structured factor in the background of opportunities and constraints that are built into mothers' daily routines (Cochran *et al.* 1993; Bell and Ribbens 1994). Webs of social ties and relationships can give mothers access to resources both materially, in terms of informal child-care support, and as systems of beliefs or moralities and shared social identities.

In Britain, there is enormous local variation in the availability, cost and quality of formal public, private and voluntary sector child-care provision (Moss 1991). The pre-school facilities that are available within any particular neighbourhood can be crucial to the social support networks into which lone mothers are linked, including their ability to draw on such networks for child care (see Bell and Ribbens 1994). For the most part, lone mothers rely on family and other neighbourhood support networks for child care (Popay and Jones 1990; Bradshaw and Millar 1991). However, local variation of formal and informal child care as a factor in lone mothers' ability to take up paid work has not been much explored. The availability of this material provision – and the circumstances under which it can be utilized – may well depend on socially created or re-created neighbourhood moral beliefs about mothers working and about lone motherhood. In turn, these beliefs may play a role in the ability of lone mothers to take up paid employment.

Transgressing the local norms or moralities may result in any available kin or friendship child-care support being withdrawn. For example, Jordan *et al.*'s (1992) study of employment decisions among white, working-class, low-income households (both couple and lone mother), living on a deprived council estate, revealed the importance of the need to comply with local neighbourhood systems of values. Economic rationality was less important than moral ideas about roles and responsibilities in mothers' uptake of paid work. While the lone mothers on the estate had a stronger desire for paid work than mothers in heterosexual couples, they were juggling this with the prevalent neighbourhood morality that mothers should prioritize caring for their own children and only 'fit in' paid work. Jordan *et al.*'s study was carried out in Exeter but, similarly, the lowest lone-mother employment rates found in Brighton and Hove include large deprived council estates, mainly housing white, working-class people. Possibly the Exeter estate's system of values also operates in estates in Brighton and Hove.

As a defining status for themselves, lone mothers can regard their situation in various ways (see Crow and Hardey 1992; Edwards and Duncan 1996), from positive to negative, from short-term to long-term. This can affect their embeddedness in particular social support networks. For example, a small-scale study in York (Edwards 1992) revealed a number of middle-class lone mothers who worked full-time utilizing formal day-care provision. They rejected the label lone parent as representing failure, tended not to mix with other lone mothers, and felt out of place with the married mothers who surrounded them in the more suburban home-owning neighbourhoods. A similar situation appears to be the case for the lone mothers we contacted in a suburban area of Brighton, such that they are not keen on taking part in research focusing on lone mothers!

Other groups of lone mothers in some neighbourhoods may value lone motherhood, and perhaps paid work, as part of alternative household daily life, stressing departure from traditional roles and independence from men. They may organize informal child care and other support networks on this basis, as Mädje and Neusüss (1994) found in an area of Berlin. Typically, these are likely to be middle-class, highly educated lone mothers living in gentrifying areas – as we are also finding in Brighton. Moreover, Gordon's (1990) study of feminist mothers in Finland and Britain, from a variety of class and ethnic backgrounds, found that lone mothers in particular were involved in local child-care groups organized by themselves.

Black lone mothers, as discussed, are more likely to view paid work and (lone) motherhood as integral. African-Caribbean women in particular are over five times more likely to be lone mothers than white women, and to be single (never married). Single mothers overall show lower rates of paid work (Bartholomew *et al.* 1992). However, black lone mothers are more likely to be economically active and much less likely to work part-time, irrespective of age and child-care responsibilities (Bruegel 1989). They also, typically, live in inner-city neighbourhoods – areas that often are in economic decline.

## LOCAL LABOUR MARKETS

Job availability is crucial, even if lone mothers want paid work and are supported in this materially and normatively. Ermisch (1991) has shown that lone mothers' employment does indeed fall in recession. Moreover, remarkably persistent horizontal and vertical occupational sex segregation, whereby women are concentrated in particular occupations and at lower status levels, means that the jobs available to women are generally the least well paid and secure (Millar and Glendinning 1989; Walby 1986). Often women's jobs are not sufficient to provide adequately for one household, especially if expensive child care also has to be bought. Moreover, black women are doubly disadvantaged in the labour market – constrained by both race and gender (Phizacklea 1982). The supply of jobs is spatially structured through local labour markets and, as with neighbour-hoods, there is considerable variability in lone mothers' employment rates at this level (taking District Councils as measuring units).[4] In 1991, the proportion of lone mothers in paid work varied from 25 per cent to 70 per cent, and from 6 per cent to 29 per cent for full-time employment. High employment areas (over 50 per cent in employment and 20 per cent full-time) included the Lancashire cotton towns and the Potteries in Staffordshire, as well as areas in the East Midlands around Northampton and Leicester, west London and parts of the so-called western crescent of recent high growth stretching around

London, from Cambridge through Berkshire to Southampton. Low employment areas (below 30 per cent in employment and 10 per cent full-time) included Merseyside, most of Wales, the North East, South Yorkshire, much of the South West and parts of East Anglia.

There are also temporal variations in the spatial patterning of lone mothers' employment. While the employment rate for lone mothers on average declined over the 1980s, this decline was especially marked in the conurbations. Elsewhere, lone mothers' employment has been more stable, fluctuating with the economic cycle (Bartholomew *et al.* 1992). This suggests that the particular features of local labour markets can also facilitate or constrain lone mothers' employment.

Mothers generally have limited job search areas because of domestic, transport and sexual harassment constraints (Pickup 1988), and these are likely to be even more severe for lone mothers. However, while lone mothers may face particular difficulties in taking up paid work, their relative propensity to take paid work varies within different areas of Britain in much the same way as it does for women as a whole. The combination of occupational gendering with spatial divisions of labour means that those areas with high rates of lone-mother employment are those areas with a tradition of women's full-time work. The Lancashire cotton towns, the Potteries and central Scotland are among the leading examples of areas where women have traditionally been seen as paid workers as much as homemakers (see Lewis 1989). Areas with no tradition of women as paid workers, often with declining labour markets, such as Merseyside, the North East and South Wales, show low employment rates (Duncan 1991a).

Yet in many of the areas most favourable for women's full-time employment, there has been economic decline. Women's participation in the cotton textiles labour force in Lancashire, for example, has always been very high, but this labour force now scarcely exists. None the less, full-time paid work by women, including lone mothers, is among the highest in the country. Conversely, some areas where there has been economic growth, such as East Anglia or parts of the western crescent, do not show a similar trend in women's employment. This suggests that regional gender divisions of labour are intimately bound up with other social changes. Women's propensity to take up paid work is not just a function of local economic structures, but reflects the way women, especially mothers, are socially integrated into society – as workers and/or homemakers. (See Duncan 1991a and Mark-Lawson 1988 for regional differences in Britain; Duncan 1991b on west inner London; Whatmore 1991 on farming areas; and Sackmann and Haüssermann 1994 on Germany.)

Thus a crucial context for lone mothers' decisions and abilities to try for paid work or not is the local 'gender contract' (Hirdmann 1990). This is a set of social expectations, discourses and possibilities, linked to the gendered material and normative moral rationalities identified above, affecting whether women are positioned locally as paid workers and/or mothers and homemakers. Cross-national differences in women's labour-force participation can also be explained in similar terms.

## NATIONAL WELFARE REGIMES

The policies that various European states adopt in relation to motherhood and paid work can be distinguished in terms of various gender contracts, embodying expectations and setting out parameters of what women and men should be, how they perceive themselves and what they do (see Duncan 1994 for a review) This explains the differences in lone mothers' employment between European countries referred to in the introduction to this chapter.

Here, we compare the policy contexts for lone mothers' employment in Germany, Sweden and Britain. These countries are archetypical cases, within Europe, of conservative, social democratic and liberal state welfare regimes (Esping-Andersen 1990).[5]

In Germany, 35 per cent of lone mothers have incomes below half the national average, while in Sweden this is just 2 per cent. In Britain, this is the case for 60 per cent of lone-mother families. This is related to the uptake of paid work. In Germany, 58 per cent of lone mothers are in paid work (35 per cent full-time), and in Sweden it is 87 per cent (54 per cent full-time, but with many 'long part-time' jobs, nearly equivalent to full-time in terms of hours worked).[6] In Britain, however, only 34 per cent of lone mothers obtain the bulk of their income from paid work, in Germany and Sweden this reached 54 per cent and 70 per cent respectively (Gustafsson and Kjulin 1991; Björnberg 1992; Roll 1992). Indicatively, and again in contrast to Britain, more German and Swedish lone mothers are in paid work, especially full-time, than partnered mothers.

In Germany, state policy positions married and cohabiting women primarily as mothers in traditional male breadwinner–female homemaker families. For partnered mothers the most rational economic decision and the most socially legitimate are the same – to become a housewife (possibly modernized by part-time work). Family wages and the tax benefit system compensate for loss of income, while child-care provision and the school system (with varying hours and no meal provision) leave little choice. Thus lone mothers do present a specific problem – the absent breadwinner role has to be filled. While means-tested lone-parent allowances are often available, grandparents or fathers are legally obliged to provide support to cover other claims on social assistance (Mädje and Neusüss 1994). In this way, lone motherhood does not seem to undermine or challenge the given gender order; rather, in reinforcing the male breadwinner role, it confirms the prevailing national gender contract.

In Sweden, the state regards lone mothers as just another type of worker, where the tax, benefit and welfare system treats all adult women as workers. These workers may also be parents, and hence the development of a pervasive child-care system and rights to parental leave and reduced working hours. Some workers, like lone mothers, may have particular problems, and so local authorities usually give them preferential treatment in child-care provision. State policy, however, does not see lone mothers as a particular social category in themselves, or as posing any overall social problem, let alone a threat to the national gender contract.

In Britain, the state ostensibly gives mothers a choice on whether to take up paid work or not. On an underlying level, though, traditional motherhood is assumed in terms of (lack of) public child-care provision, which is among the lowest in Europe, but not in terms of family wages. Thus it is difficult for mothers to participate on equal terms with men, and with other women, in the labour market, but paradoxically they need to. Policies thus reinforce mothers' employment in part-time jobs, which are often low paid, insecure and sometimes even without employment rights and protection. Lone mothers are particularly disadvantaged, with as many as 50 per cent having no access to any sort of child care (Popay and Jones 1990; Bradshaw and Millar 1991). Mothers are implicitly dependent on a male breadwinner or, if this fails as with lone mothers, on increasingly minimal and stigmatized state benefits.

This situation leads to lone mothers in Britain being regarded as, at best, a social problem or, at worst, a threat to the social order. There is ambiguity regarding women's integration into the social order, whether as workers in the labour market (as in Sweden) or as mothers and housewives in families (as in Germany). If the state provides sufficient child-care support, then it implicitly takes the position that all mothers are primarily workers. If it treats all mothers primarily as homemakers, this also costs an awful lot, even at minimal levels. Both political strategies risk offending powerful interest groups and alienating voters, and are fraught with political implications *vis-à-vis* the relations between men and women and the nature of 'the family'.

## CONCLUSION: LINKING THE CONTEXTS

The apparent irrationality of British lone mothers' decreasing employment rates over the past two decades, unlike married mothers in Britain and also lone mothers in most of western Europe, is related to other shifts in addition to changes in the labour market and benefit structures. There have been two main, and interlocking, shifts in child-care availability and in gendered moral rationalities.

First, in the 1970s the higher percentage of lone mothers in paid work was matched by the majority of them living in multi-unit households, most usually their own parents' home, and with their own mothers' (grandmothers) providing child care (Land 1993) – following traditional familial moral obligations. Grandmothers are now far more likely to be in paid work themselves, and do not always wish to undertake such caring (see, for example, Cotterill 1994).

Second, in the 1970s lone mothers formed a smaller overall proportion of families. They either continued within the dominant gendered morality for motherhood – widows for whom the state substituted the deceased's breadwinner role – or fell outside it – they had children out of wedlock. To be a single mother was to be in a marginal and stigmatized position and, therefore, not subject to another dominant norm of 'normal' motherhood, that of full-time homemaker. As lone mothers have become an increasing proportion of the population, and as the situation has become one that 'normal' mothers may face (especially given the rise in divorce and separation), so they too become subject to dominant understandings of mothers and their role.

However, conceptions of motherhood, in relation to its incorporation of paid work, can vary between different social groups of lone mothers, often living in particular neighbourhoods. Moreover, while similar developments in the proportions of lone mothers have taken place elsewhere in western Europe, there have not been similar declines in their employment rates. Different national gender contracts have meant other welfare regimes have either recognized these changes (as in Sweden, with child care) or absorbed them (as in Germany).

Paradoxically, as lone mothers have become numerically more important and have been incorporated into dominant norms for motherhood, discourses around lone motherhood have become heavily politicized in Britain. Dominant discourses impose definitions of what lone mothers are and what they should do, and also have very practical consequences in influencing policies and hence the provision of resources. Similarly, gender divisions of labour operate differentially at the level of local labour markets, reflecting the interaction of spatial divisions of capitalist labour with regional views of the gender contract. It is not only particular jobs (especially socially defined women's jobs) that will be differentially distributed but also conceptions as to whether women are mothers and/or workers. Lone mothers' job opportunities and their propensity to take up paid work will be locally differentiated. At the level of social networks and neighbourhoods, lone mothers' access to resources in terms of child care and social support will vary in interaction with local and social group-based discourses and socially held moral rationalities about (lone) motherhood and paid work.

It is in these interacting contexts that lone mothers take decisions about paid work. For instance, the existence of social networks and support at a neighbourhood level, and how these may constrain or offer opportunities to lone mothers, may be related to differences in the national welfare state regime. Where countries have developed policies that favour high levels of mothers' employment combined with high levels of provision of formal child care, the development of local support networks among women may be less likely. In Sweden, Scott (1982) suggests that self-help autonomous networks among women are rare because the government has incorporated feminism. Conversely, where policies do not support mothers' employment or child-care provision, local social networks may play a stronger part. In Germany, Epstein et al. (1986) found that women had a sense of belonging to a specifically female culture and holding family-based values, with German governments also emphasizing traditional family life through welfare policies. In Britain, informal networks of women are significant in child care.

As we have argued, there is a risk in over-stressing the supremacy of welfare state regimes and also of individualistic economic calculations. Too often both are seen as all-determining, so that the complexity of lone mothers' responses to the structures in which they live is not allowed for. Viewing lone mothers as women in social context, rather than as 'rational economic man', allows us to see beyond the passive respondents in a simple stimulus–response policy model. It allows us to see lone mothers as participating women, socially creating and shaping opportunities for themselves and their children, acting within the constraints and opportunities provided by different social contexts.

## ACKNOWLEDGEMENTS

Our thanks to Rob Eastwood, whose comments on our ideas concerning the gendered nature of economic and moral rationalities were invaluable.

## NOTES

1  In this assumption, personal welfare, or economic well-being or utility, is usually defined as monetary income and leisure. The notion of leisure is particularly problematic in relation to women (see, for example, Wimbush and Talbot 1988).
2  Our research is funded by the Economic and Social Research Council under grant number R000234960. As it is still in its early stages we do not draw on it extensively here. Full results from the study will be available in Duncan and Edwards (1997 forthcoming). Vignettes of lone mothers in the text are based on data from interviews carried out during the summer of 1994.
3  This can work the other way around, however. Lone mothers may undertake paid work in order to afford good quality day care (Edwards 1993).
4  District Councils (DCs) are more suitable in representing local labour markets for lone mothers than the conventionally designated Travel to Work Areas. Lone mothers, like women generally, display much shorter journeys to work than men (Flowerdew and Green 1993).
5  Esping-Andersen's work has been subject to considerable criticism by feminist researchers because of its gender blindness. None the less, these three countries would still be archetypal in the various alternative classifications proposed (see Duncan 1996).
6  In particular, parents of pre-school children have the right to a shortened working day.

# Chapter 7

# 'Parental responsibility': the reassertion of private patriarchy?

*Lorraine M. Fox Harding*

Since 1979, the Conservative governments in Britain have developed an interest in the issue of family responsibility, notably as it impinges on the scope of state responsibility and in particular on the amount of *expenditure* involved. A rhetoric of family behaviour has been developed in which certain themes, such as individual responsibility and the undesirability of dependence on the state, have become central to the aim of restoring or revitalizing family responsibility. A major preoccupation has been the area of *parental* responsibility. The Conservative interest bears the mark of a lobby known variously as neo-traditionalist, moral, and 'family values'. This lobby is internally heterogeneous, but shares a concern with the decline of the marriage-based family. A central preoccupation is the problem for government and society of the rise in lone-parent families, especially where mother-headed. For this group, the dependence of mothers on the state must be avoided. Dependence on the family, particularly for financial support, is regarded as vastly preferable.

This chapter focuses on the Child Support Act 1991 and its effects.[1] This covers resistance from men, reactions from women, government responses to the dissatisfaction with the Act, and likely continued dissatisfaction in the future. Two concepts are explored: 'parental responsibility' and 'private patriarchy'. 'Parental responsibility' can be understood in different ways, but it is clear that the government's main concern has been to shift responsibility away from the state. 'Private patriarchy' refers to the form of patriarchy where women are controlled by, and dependent on, individual patriarchs in a household. Since the late nineteenth century this form of patriarchy has been in decline in Britain as women have entered the public arena. The argument is developed along three dimensions:

1  the rejection of private patriarchy by women;
2  the rejection of private patriarchy by men; and
3  the particular type of private patriarchy that the Child Support Act may recreate in the short and long term.

I argue that while the Act may appear to be attempting to reinstate a form of private patriarchy in the sense of making more women economically dependent on individual men, it appears more strongly to be part of a project of rolling back the state. In this light I consider the extent to which the Act is anti-women, anti-men, anti-child and anti-family.

The Child Support Act 1991 was the product of some rapid developments in the late 1980s and early 1990s that focused specifically on the cost to the public purse of the growing numbers of single-parent families in receipt of state cash benefits.[2] The steeply rising costs occurred not only because the total group of single parents had increased but also because the composition of that group had changed.[3] There were more lone parents without maintenance and more who were never-married mothers. The government produced its proposals in a White Paper, *Children Come First* (Lord Chancellor *et al.* 1990), towards the end of 1990, and after the briefest of consultation exercises the ensuing Child Support Act passed through all its stages and was on the statute book by July 1991. This was a truly astonishing speed.

The Child Support Act's main provisions relate to how maintenance from an 'absent parent', usually but not invariably the father, whether ever married to the child's mother or not, shall be calculated and enforced. The Act set up an administrative agency called the Child Support Agency to assess and enforce child-maintenance liability. This agency largely supersedes the role of the courts in this area. The Act deploys a complex and rigid formula to determine the amount of maintenance.[4] Where parents who have care of a child are receiving one of three types of means-tested benefit – income support, family credit, disability working allowance – they are required, on pain of a financial penalty, to co-operate in the search for the absent parent.[5] Other parents with care who wish to enforce a maintenance liability have to make use of the Agency; they cannot go through the courts.

A crucial aspect of the Act, and one that makes the government's underlying intention of reducing its benefits bill only too clear, is that the parents with care who are on income support have their maintenance payments wholly offset against their income support entitlement – that is, income support is reduced pound for pound of maintenance. So payment of maintenance by the erstwhile partner, while saving government money, will leave the parent with care no better off. Parents with care who are on family credit and disability working allowance *are* allowed to benefit by a small amount.[6] It is clear that the government's intention here is to encourage single mothers into full-time work. The absent parents are thus paying their money to benefit the Treasury, not their children and the parent with care. This means that there is no *positive* incentive for absent parents to pay, or for parents with care on income support to seek to have them pay. The inducements are all negative. It can reasonably be argued that many informal arrangements between separated parents are likely to be upset by the workings of the Act.

It should be noted that the construction of parental responsibility within the Child Support Act is entirely financial, and is independent of marriage. It is also independent of any consideration of what the actual relationship between biological parents was. A rapist, a casual sexual partner, or a sperm donor in a private arrangement are all potentially financially liable parents for the purposes of the Act (Department of Social Security 1993b). The government's overriding aim is clearly to reduce social security costs by recouping more maintenance. Another aim is to reduce benefit costs by encouraging more lone mothers into the labour market, by enlarging the scope of family credit and in some ways making it more favourable than income support. This contradicts the views of the neo-traditionalist or 'family values' lobby on the importance of mothers in domestic family settings for the rearing of children.

## THE CHILD SUPPORT ACT: EFFECTS AND REACTIONS

Initially, parents with care with new or changed claims for the three benefits mentioned (income support, family credit, and disability working allowance) were subject to the Act's provisions, as well as parents with care not on these benefits but without an existing maintenance order or agreement. Existing claimants of the relevant benefits are to be brought into the net gradually, while non-benefit cases *with* existing maintenance agreements or orders are not allowed to use the agency until April 1996. Soon after the beginning of implementation in April 1993, considerable resistance to the provisions of the Act was in evidence.

Reaction from male absent parents became apparent in the media from the summer of 1993. Men spoke to the media, contacted their MPs, and formed campaigns. The issues they were concerned with included: the amounts of money demanded; the Agency pursuit of men who were already paying maintenance under court-approved settlements (some thought that only 'feckless' fathers who had paid nothing would be pursued); and the fact that the Agency was taking no account of existing 'clean-break' or no-maintenance deals in which men had often handed over their share of the matrimonial property. The formula also did not take account of the costs of contact between the absent parent and the children, nor of any exceptional costs the absent parent might have, such as those associated with disability. It was argued that the Agency's operations were upsetting existing arrangements between separated parents. The facts that the Act operated retrospectively and that stepchildren were not allowable for were particularly resented. It was argued that the Agency was directing its energies at easily traceable, 'soft' targets. The protesters were, perhaps, disproportionately employed and middle class. Campaigns were launched and public demonstrations took place.

While men were vocal in their objections to the Child Support Act, at first relatively little was heard of women's reactions. The Child Poverty Action Group was concerned that women did not want to bring their cases forward, and therefore certain issues were not being aired in the media (Garnham and Knights 1994). The Agency was reported as saying that many mothers were delighted. However, the Campaign Against the Child Support Act was concerned about women being intimidated by the Agency to give the names of absent parents, and intimate questions being asked about their sex lives where paternity was denied. It seemed that in some cases there was violence, and that some men who had previously acknowledged paternity were now denying it. There were also concerns about the loss or reduction of income support when maintenance was ordered but then fell into default. There were particular problems in assessing accurately the income of absent parents who were self-employed. The reduction of income support pound for pound as maintenance was paid was a particular issue for concern. Research by Clarke et al. (1994b) showed that in a group of over fifty mothers on income-related benefits, none was better off, and some (13 per cent) were worse off, as a result of the Act. Informal arrangements were adversely affected, and conflict between former partners intensified, sometimes with effects on the children.

Under pressure from MPs, the Commons Select Committee on Social Security, and others, the government modified the formula slightly in February 1994. But it still did not allow for the cost of stepchildren, nor did it take account of clean-break settlements. Some major grievances remained unaddressed, and dissaffection continued. In 1994 the situation was being kept under review. In July, management consultants were sent in to review the Child Support Agency, and in September its Chief Executive resigned after apologizing for 'performance failure'. Extra money and staff were allocated. In November 1994 the House of Commons Select Committee again made recommendations for change, but disagreed on whether there should be a disregard of maintenance for those on income support.

## THE LIKELY LONG-TERM EFFECTS OF THE CHILD SUPPORT ACT

Within the current rules, many absent parents will continue to face maintenance demands far in excess of their previous payments, and an increasing number of absent parents will be brought into the operations of the Agency. The long-term reduction of income for absent parents and their existing families will progressively erode their standard of living. This will probably result in strain and relationship breakdown. Relationships and arrangements between absent and caring parents also seem likely to face further problems. It may reasonably be predicted that as the number of affected absent parents increases, and their grievances do not go away, they will become more organized, and will learn to campaign more assertively against the Act. Offsetting this it may also be that a degree of accommodation will take place, with absent parents adapting in various ways to the Agency's demands. Perhaps some sort of cultural shift will take place in popular concepts and expectations of absent parents' roles and responsibilities, away from notions of clean breaks or uncommitted fatherhood, towards ideas of ongoing financial responsibility for biological children regardless of the status of the relationship between the parents. However, this seems to go against current trends in relationships between men and women in the United Kingdom.

Concerning the reactions of parents with care, those parents who are not on income support will in time stand to make a real gain in income in some cases. In particular, those with earnings that take them above the family credit level may find that, with the addition of maintenance from the other parent, they are appreciably better-off. From 1996, parents with care on better incomes are likely to feature increasingly among the Agency's clientele. There may at that point be something of a groundswell of support for the Act. But parents with care on the means-tested benefits may still actually be worse-off in real terms, or suffer in other ways.

As has been argued, the primary objective of government in passing the Child Support Act was to make public expenditure savings in social security, mainly by removing significant numbers of lone parents from income support. However, savings may be smaller than anticipated. This is because current high levels of unemployment and the absence of free or subsidized child care make it difficult for lone mothers to move into employment. Unemployment also affects absent parents. The Child Support Agency itself, of course, carries a cost to run.

At this stage it remains difficult to assess what precisely the net savings of the Act will be. The Agency's targets were not met in its first year.

## CONCEPTS RELEVANT TO THE CHILD SUPPORT ACT

Two concepts will now be examined as relevant to a wider understanding of the Act. The first is the government's understanding of the notion of 'parental responsibility'. The second may be seen as another way of interpreting the first, and this is the concept of 'private patriarchy'. The latter will be discussed with particular reference to Sylvia Walby's work (1990).

### Parental responsibility

The principle of 'parental responsibility' is found in the Child Support Act, also in the Children Act 1989 and the Criminal Justice Act 1991. Edwards and Halpern (1992) argue that the parental responsibility concept is a central theme underpinning recent legislation on children's welfare and their financial support, and children's criminality. They suggest that the concept creates a suitable moral climate in which various policy changes can be justified. While the different types of parental responsibility present in the three Acts – the Children Act, Child Support Act and Criminal Justice Act – are not always consistent, the concept is 'used as a powerful instrument of social policy in shaping the family' (Edwards and Halpern 1992: 118). It promotes parental responsibility in place of state responsibility, a position that is sustained by *laissez-faire* ideology, although it is also – inconsistently with *laissez-faire* – a mechanism of greater state control.

It can be argued, then, that the government is using the notion of parental responsibility in a unified way. The concept meshes with a wider strategy for broader family responsibility, more private dependency, and fewer state-dependent families. It may be noted that the Children Act 1989 did not originate in a desire to expand parental responsibility as the government defines and values it, nor is the Act only about this. But certain elements in the Act tend in this direction. The principle of minimum intervention set out in Section 1(5) states that a court may not make any order regarding a child unless satisfied that this is a better outcome for the child than no order. Such a principle, alongside the definition of parents as having responsibilities rather than rights in Sections 2 and 3, highlights the government's aim of leaving more responsibility to parents and less to the state. Parental responsibility cannot be surrendered, and can only be transferred following a court hearing. 'Absent parents' who have once been married do not lose parental responsibility. Unmarried fathers can achieve it by order or agreement (Section 4). As I have commented elsewhere, 'In a sense the Children Act has been "used". The vastness of the Act, the debates that focused on other important sections, enabled the parental responsibility and non-intervention sections to pass with, perhaps, less scrutiny than they deserved' (Fox Harding 1994: 102).

The Criminal Justice Act 1991, on the other hand, makes parents more accountable for their children's criminal behaviour. Looking at parental responsibility in the three Acts, Edwards and Halpern (1992) identify three major, not always consistent, threads:

1  responsibility that emphasizes an emotional and psychological commitment,
2  financial responsibility (*to* the state, *for* children),
3  blame for a failure of parental responsibility which contributes to delinquency.

It is the second of these, financial responsibility, but not necessarily the other two, that is relevant to the Child Support Act. Parental financial responsibility is widened. Other measures also in effect increase the financial burdens of parenthood, while reducing the cost of young people to the state: for example, the removal of income support rights for 16- to 17-year-olds.

Eekelaar (1991) has also explored the notion of parental responsibility, in relation to the Children Act. He argues that parental responsibility here can represent two ideas:

1 Parents must behave dutifully to their children.
2 Responsibility for child care belongs to parents rather than the state.

It is the second idea, of parental rather than state responsibility, that, Eekelaar maintains, came to be dominant during the development of the Children Act. It rests upon an ideology 'which identifies the legal concept of parental responsibility with a perception about the ordering of relationships in the natural world' (Eekelaar 1991: 37). This ideology has led to a weakening of the state's supervisory role in relation to parent–child relationships. Eekelaar argues that the expression 'parental responsibility' changed its function over the 1980s, and a slippage occurred from responsibility 1 to responsibility 2. The first refers to parental behaviour towards the child, the second to the role exercised by the parent as opposed to someone else. In the Children Act the shift from responsibility in the first sense, dutiful behaviour, to responsibility in the second, parents rather than the state, is shown by a number of instances. First, parental responsibility is pre-eminently individual responsibility rather than lying with state institutions; and second, parental responsibility may not be voluntarily surrendered to the state; while third, parental responsibility remains undiminished even when child care is 'shared' with the state. The fourth point is that parental responsibility cannot be surrendered or transferred to another individual; and the fifth that there is a general weakening of state power and control over parental conduct. Eekelaar points out, with relation to the fourth point of non-surrenderability, that parental responsibilities under the Children Act endure with more tenacity than parental rights and duties under the previous scheme. Responsibility is retained by both parents after divorce, for example. A parent cannot divest himself or herself of the legal responsibility of his or her parenthood *even through the agency of a court order*' (Eekelaar 1991: 43, italics in the original).

In the context of the Child Support Act, the state appears more closely involved in parental duties, but only in specifying more strongly how financial obligations should be met. This is being done with the aim of shifting the costs of children away from the state and back to individuals. The state is supervising more closely in order to shed a responsibility. Thus there is an increase in state control, not of the way parents behave to their children in a general sense but only of how much absent parents pay out. The state is then withdrawing from its responsibilities, not its power. And the financial responsibility of biological parenthood may not be voluntarily surrendered under the Act, even if the offer were made to surrender all 'parental rights' with it. The only way out for a parent wishing to absolve himself or herself of the financial obligations of parenthood would be via the child's adoption by another party, or via a denial of biological parenthood. Parental responsibility in the Act is thus tenacious, and this is regardless of marriage or anything else regarding the relationship between the two biological parents. In this sense the Act is innovative, as family law *has* hitherto made distinctions between children on the grounds of their parents' legal relationship.

### 'Private patriarchy' and the Child Support Act

Walby (1990) has explored a general movement away from 'private patriarchy' in women's position in society. She comments that recent British history has seen a change in both the degree and form of patriarchy, with reductions in some specific aspects, but also counter-attack, often on new issues. Thus she argues that private patriarchy has given way to public patriarchy, and distinguishes between the two as follows:

> Private patriarchy is based upon household production, with a patriarch controlling women individually and directly in the relatively private sphere of the home. Public patriarchy is based on structures other than the household, ... institutions conventionally regarded as part of the public domain are central in the maintenance of patriarchy.
>
> (Walby 1990: 178)

In private patriarchy it is the individual man as husband/father who subordinates the woman, and women are excluded from the public sphere. In public patriarchy, women have access to both public and private arenas, but are subordinated within both. Women's subordination is carried out by men acting collectively, although the household may remain a site of oppression for women as well. With the movement from private to public patriarchy, women have been segregated in, rather than excluded from, paid work. They have been less confined to the household than they were. They have been subordinated in, rather than excluded from, cultural institutions, and subjected to sexual controls in the public arena rather than from a specific husband. Women's exclusion from the state gave way to their subordination in the state. Walby considers that, in Britain, the height of the private form of patriarchy was found in the mid-nineteenth century in the middle classes, among whom women were largely excluded from the public sphere in which many new bases of power for men were developing. Since then, and partly as a result of the successes of first-wave feminism, there has been a reduction in some forms of oppression and a movement towards the public form of patriarchy, with women, including married women, entering the public sphere, for example paid work, but being subordinated there. Marriages (the 'private' sphere) are more easily dissolved, although women remain responsible for child care, often under conditions of poverty. After the Second World War, women's access to waged labour and to state social security payments expanded, effectively freeing them further from marriage. Walby, writing at the end of the 1980s, considered that we had not yet seen the full development of the trend towards a more public form of patriarchy.

But the state is itself patriarchal. On the question of lone mothers, Walby comments:

> While they lose their own individual patriarch, they do not lose their subordination to other patriarchal structures and practices. Indeed they become even more exposed to certain of the more diffused public sets of patriarchal practices.
>
> (Walby 1990: 197)

Thus the lone mother's income level and standard of living are determined no longer primarily by her husband but either by the patriarchal state or by the patriarchally structured labour market. It is the state and the market rather than the private patriarch that determine her life. 'She substitutes public for private patriarchy' (Walby 1990: 197).

The significance of the shift from private to public patriarchy for a discussion of the Child Support Act is that the Act is attempting to reverse recent historical trends in which women have moved from confinement to and dependence on the private sphere to a subordinated position within the public sphere. Women as parents have become increasingly dependent on a collectivized system for provision for economic survival, that is social security, and on the labour market; and correspondingly they have become less dependent on the financial support of individual men. The Child Support Act quite specifically aims to reverse the latter trend, while encouraging lone mothers further into the labour market as well. Three aspects of private patriarchy are relevant in this context: the rejection of private patriarchy by women; its rejection by men; and the type of private patriarchy that the Act is likely to reassert.

Concerning the rejection of private patriarchy by women, evidence that it is women who have resisted and overturned the extremes of private patriarchy may be found in the record of first-wave feminist campaigns to gain access for women to the public sphere (Walby 1990). Inter-war or welfare feminism was particularly concerned with expanding welfare state provisions that would benefit women (Walby 1990; Williams 1989). Second-wave feminism appearing in the 1960s was *inter alia* concerned with the importance for women of moving beyond the narrow and confining role of 'housewife' (for example, Friedan 1963). The increase in divorce since the 1960s, and the fact that over 70 per cent of divorce petitioners are women (*Social Trends* various years), along with increased numbers of women cohabiting, and producing children without either marriage or cohabitation (Joshi 1989; Kiernan and Wicks 1990; Elliott 1991; recent editions of *Social Trends*), may also be pointed to as evidence of women's 'escape' from private patriarchy, their rejection of life in households with men. It has been more possible for women to do this as other alternatives such as work and access to social security have become increasingly available. As Walby (1990: 84) comments: 'Given my argument that women get a raw deal in marriage, we would expect the propensity of women to live in marriages to decline the more that they have other alternatives.'

The problem is that the meaning of these trends is ambiguous for women. For one thing, divorce and other forms of lone parenthood, as Walby fully acknowledges, often lead to a life of poverty on low wages or benefits (Burghes 1993). The Child Support Act reflects a concern about the dependence on benefits but not necessarily about poverty as such. It attempts to make women dependent on individual men again, but not necessarily better off. A related problem is that it is not clear how far single-person/lone-parent living and independence from men represent a positive choice for women. Is it in fact men who have deliberately moved away from private patriarchy? This is the second point to be considered.

In the discussion of the rejection of private patriarchy by men, two authors quoted by Walby are relevant to the notion that men have also resisted the strictures of private patriarchy. These are Brown (1981) and Ehrenreich (1983), who suggest a reduction in commitment to the family on the part of men. Brown examines the relationship between children and parents over the last century or more and the shift from father custody to mother custody when relationships end. It seems 'natural' today that mothers keep the children on marriage break-down, yet this is a recent phenomenon. She explains this mainly in terms of the declining value of children as an economic asset (labour) due to extended education and the development of capitalism. Children have become a costly burden, an obligation. As fathers no longer benefited from children in the same way as they had, they were happy to let custody go to mothers. Custody shifted from father-right to mother-obligation. At the same time, women are increasingly under the control of public patriarchy. Significantly in the light of the passing of the Child Support Act in Britain a decade later, Brown comments on the increase of the power of higher-level, ruling-class men, over all women within public patriarchy, and the decrease of the power of lower-level men over any women. However, the main point relates to the decline of private, family patriarchy and of its value for men. Men are more able to cut their losses and meet their needs elsewhere when the benefits of being a private patriarch fail. Along similar lines, Ehrenreich (1983) suggests that men have since the 1950s revolted against the situation where they are the source of economic maintenance for women and children. For men, families became a responsibility rather than an asset. The focus of Ehrenreich's book is the ideology surrounding the breadwinner ethic and how it collapsed over the thirty years between the early 1950s and the early 1980s.

Following these arguments, the decline of marriage, the increase in less committed and less long-term sexual relationships, and the rise of lone motherhood, reflect preferences on the part of men. Some aspects of private patriarchy have perhaps proved onerous to men, and they have taken advantage of the movement of women into the public sphere to abandon their role as individual 'patriarchs'. This tendency has perhaps been exacerbated by some demands from women for greater equality within marriage, and an increase in the responsibilities and financial burdens of parenthood. It is the case that men have increasingly disappeared from the parent–child unit, whether after separation or divorce or because they were never part of this unit in the first place; and various studies have shown that they tend to lose contact with their children after divorce (Wallerstein and Blakeslee 1989).

Both the moral lobby (Dennis and Erdos 1992) and the government have been concerned about the decreasing involvement of fathers in families. The Child Support Act represents a rather drastic and clumsy attempt to halt this movement away from fathering. On a strict biological interpretation of parenthood, as found in the Act, men acquire lasting parental (financial) responsibility not only from marriage or cohabitation but from any sexual relationship that leads to a birth (unless the child is adopted) including the very casual and tenuous. The fact that some men seem to be denying paternity in an attempt to avoid maintenance payments is but one indicator that this view of parenthood is not universally shared.

Following the Child Support Act it is now more difficult for men to evade financial responsibility for children. But it may be that the government stress on such parental responsibility and the exertions of the Child Support Agency will induce men to retreat even further from the disadvantaging status of parenthood by evasion, disappearance, denial of paternity, or by attempting to ensure that paternity does not follow from sex.

In this context, what can be said of the re-creation of 'private patriarchy' by the Child Support Act? The Act will not straightforwardly re-create or reassert the private patriarchy of earlier times. Lone mothers are not being forced or explicitly pressured to form households with the men who are the fathers of their children, or even with other men. The type of private patriarchy that the Child Support Act is endeavouring to reinstate is a financial dependence of lone parents (mothers) on absent biological parents (fathers). It is dependence as far as the mothers are concerned, and responsibility as far as the fathers are concerned. Mothers are not being required to 'do anything in return' for this support – to provide services for the men, live with them, or allow them greater access to the children, although some men may well seek some returns. And the maintenance will in principle be enforceable as a legal right. In that sense it is only a partial private patriarchy that is being sought. Also some women will resist pursuing fathers for maintenance notwithstanding the benefit penalty (Child Poverty Action Group 1993b), and so will avoid private patriarchy, at a price.

Furthermore, the reinstitution of this type of partial private patriarchy has quite clearly come from that embodiment of public patriarchy, the state. It may be seen as an expression of public patriarchy that a male-dominated government and legislature should pass an Act reducing female dependence on public funds and increasing such dependence on private sources and individual men. Men acting collectively have been moving to shift a perceived burden onto some men as individuals. The (mis)perception that the Child Support Act would only adversely affect 'feckless' men who paid little or nothing facilitated this political aim. Also, some of the Act's explicit, albeit subsidiary, agenda is to encourage lone mothers into the labour force. This is an encouragement of an alternative form of public patriarchy: women should gain their livelihood from selling their labour in a male-dominated labour market, as a preferable alternative to claiming state benefits. This would therefore not constitute a reassertion of private patriarchy.

What of the longer-term effects? As a result of the Child Support Act, will women take even greater precautions against pregnancy with a non-committed partner, will they make more efforts to remain with a partner they already have when he is the father of their children, will men be more cautious about casual sex, and will they feel a firmer commitment to remaining with a partner who is the mother of their children, and with the children? If such trends become noticeable – and these aims could well be part of a hidden agenda in the Act – then private patriarchy will be strengthened in a more general sense. That is, women will in practice be more subject to the control of individual patriarchs than they have been in the recent past. On the other hand, men's 'flight from fatherhood' may be intensified.

## CONCLUSION

The Child Support Act appears to be part of a project of rolling back the state rather than an attempt to invoke parental responsibility or private patriarchy as such. Men are being told to pay more and lone mothers are being forced into greater financial dependence on individual men, but mothers are also being encouraged – or pressured – into the labour market. The primary concern is to get lone mothers *off the state's back*. The Child Support Act, it is argued, is about 'less state responsibility' (Eekelaar 1991). But I maintain that the Act does have important implications for both parental responsibility and private patriarchy, as I analyse it in relation to women, men, children and families.

Is the Child Support Act anti-feminist and anti-women? The adverse effects for women are greater dependence on individual men, possibly more control by men, and possibly loss of income in cash and/or kind due to a combination of factors. A reversion to a degree of private patriarchy conflicts with feminist aims. The beneficial effects for women include raised income for some, and perhaps easing of the path into employment. Also in the category of adversely affected women are those whose present partner is an absent parent in relation to someone else. Some of these second families will experience, and are already experiencing, a dramatic drop in standard of living. In some cases, second wives or partners are being expected to contribute indirectly to the maintenance of their partner's former family.

Is the Child Support Act anti-men? Absent fathers in work are experiencing marked loss of income and are protesting bitterly. Some clearly feel a sharp sense of injustice. However, some in the stepfather category who do not have children of their own in another household may experience an easing of their circumstances, with raised main-tenance payments for their stepchildren coming into the household.

Is the Child Support Act anti-child? Absent so far from this discussion is the child as a separate entity. One aspect of the Act that has been defended is its role in making more open the actual financial costs of raising a child. Some maintenance awards under the old court-based system were absurdly low in relation to the true cost of child maintenance. The needs of children are thus more explicitly asserted. Nevertheless some children will undoubtedly suffer, chiefly those in the various types of household where income drops, and those who have reduced contact with their absent parent because he or she feels financially unable to visit them, have them to stay, and take part in other aspects of the parental role. Conversely, some absent parents may demand contact where it has not occurred before (maintenance payments can be reduced where children stay with the absent parent part of the time), and this will not necessarily be in the child's interests. Conflicts between adults, possibly involving violence, are likely to affect the children.

Is the Child Support Act anti-family? Relationships may be put under strain by the Act and its provisions. These include relationships between former partners whose existing arrangements and agree-ments are disrupted, and relationships between present partners where maintenance payments to a former partner create financial stress, or where, for example, the Agency's inquiries bring to light the existence of an extra-marital child. It cannot be determined at the time of writing whether these stresses will feed into further separation or divorce and family violence, but they may well do so. The short-term priority of the Act is not to strengthen or facilitate family relationships but to raise money. However, there is the possibility that it will produce more cautious and more committed, rather than just more inescapable, relationships in the future. Conversely, it may encourage men to fly further from commitment, because the responsibilities of non-resident fatherhood have become more onerous. Other overall effects on 'the family', as an institution with diverse forms, are yet to be seen.

## NOTES ON CHANGES IN 1994/5

This chapter reflects the position on the Child Support Act as it was in autumn 1994. However, important concessions were made by the government in December 1994 and early in 1995. Briefly, these changes were, first, that action would be deferred on certain categories of cases (where parents had not co-operated or supplied enough information, where they were receiving income support – without change in their claim – before April 1993, or where they were not on benefit at all). This was said to be a 'reprieve' for about 300,000 absent fathers (*Guardian*, 21 December 1994). Second, no absent parent would have to pay more than 30 per cent of his or her net income in maintenance and the maximum maintenance amount would be reduced; absent parents would be able to apply to a Tribunal for a departure from the formula in exceptional circumstances, such as high expenses connected with travel to work or disability; some allowance would be made for clean-break settlements where property or capital was involved; and some allowance would be made for the absent parent's stepchildren's and new partner's housing costs. Most of these changes favoured absent parents. However, a 'back to work bonus' was offered to parents with care on benefit who found employment; parents with care would also be able to appeal the maintenance assessment; and where their maintenance payments decreased as a result of the changes, certain means-tested benefits (family credit and disability working allowance) would be adjusted partially (but only partially) in the short term (as well as fully in the long term), to take account of this (Wylie 1995). A White Paper, *Improving Child Support*, set out the proposals. The changes were to be phased in gradually. The concessions to absent parents on the whole reduce fathers' liabilities to maintain, and therefore possibly mothers' incomes, depending on their benefit situation. However, the much more limited concessions to parents with care might offset this.

At this stage it is not possible to judge the overall effects of the changes, but the emergence of more 'loopholes' may weaken any attempted restoration of private patriarchy through the Child Support Act.

## NOTES

1  This chapter reflects the position on the Child Support Act as it was in the autumn of 1994.
2  For example, in 1979, there were around 830,000 lone parents in Great Britain, some 38 per cent of whom (318,000) were receiving the then Supplementary Benefit (Child Poverty Action Group 1990); by 1993 there were around 1.3 million, about three-quarters of whom (nearly a million) were on income support (Child Poverty Action Group 1993a). The income support bill for lone parents was almost £2 billion in 1988–9. Total social security expenditure on lone parents was nearly double this amount (National Audit Office 1990). The numbers and proportion of lone mothers receiving child maintenance had declined (National Audit Office 1990). By 1989 only 30 per cent of lone mothers received regular child maintenance (Lord Chancellor et al. 1990).
3  The trends included not only a growth in the number of lone parents overall but an expansion, within this total, in the number of never-married mothers specifically. Other factors contributing to rising costs were: a decreased tendency on the part of the Department of Health and Security, later the Department of Social Security, to pursue liable fathers for contributions when single mothers claimed benefits (National Audit Office 1990); changed practice on maintenance in the courts (clean breaks); and, probably, high levels of unemployment affecting both the single parents' ability to be independent of benefits and the absent parent's ability to pay maintenance (National Audit Office 1990).
4  The formula that the Child Support Agency uses to calculate maintenance liability has been controversial, and its severity caused some surprise when it was first published, with unfavourable comparison being made with the Wisconsin scheme that was one of the government's models. Some of the effects of the formula will be commented on later in this chapter. Broadly, the amount deemed necessary to support child and parent with care, the 'maintenance bill', is determined with reference to the level of income support benefit rates. An amount known as 'exempt income' for living costs, also largely according to income support rates, is calculated for the absent parent, leaving his or her so-called assessable income; and 50 per cent of *that* is taken by the Agency until the 'maintenance bill' is paid. Once it is paid, a further 25 per cent of assessable income is taken, up to a ceiling. The assessable income of the parent with care is also a factor. The exempt income formula allows for the absent parent's existing commitments, but not totally; stepchildren by a second partnership, for example, are not counted, nor are the new partner's share of the housing costs. However, a further formula, the 'protected income', should prevent the absent parent

and his or her household from falling below the income support level themselves, thus it was hoped to lessen the incentive to give up employment in order to avoid the Child Support Agency's demands. It should be noted that the 'protected income' takes the new partner's income into account, effectively making her or him liable for maintenance for the first family. Various sanctions, including attachment of earnings and ultimately imprisonment, are available to ensure that maintenance payments are made. Even those absent parents on income support themselves because of unemployment will, if they have no children in their current household, have a small amount (slightly over £2) deducted from their weekly benefit towards the maintenance bill.

5  Failure to co-operate would usually be punished by a reduction in benefit for a time, £9.14 weekly for six months and £4.57 weekly for a further twelve months (1994 figures), unless the parent with care can show that 'harm or undue distress' (Section 6), such as violence, would occur to her or him or the children by the pursuit of the other parent for maintenance. It must be noted that this pressure, backed by a financial sanction, is applied to families who are on the means-tested state minima already, and therefore living at a low material standard (Oldfield and Yu 1993). This was a controversial aspect of the Act. It has been felt that in some cases lone parents may have valid reasons for not wishing to enforce the financial responsibilities of the other parent, and yet they may be financially disadvantaged by taking this position.

6  This is a 'disregard' of maintenance of £15, although parents on family credit, unlike those on income support, cannot have their full benefit entitlement guaranteed while the Agency receives the maintenance money and stands the loss should the absent parent default. Family credit also carries other disadvantages, such as not contributing at all towards mortgage costs.

# Chapter 8

# Social anxieties about lone motherhood and ideologies of the family

## Two sides of the same coin

*Mary McIntosh*

Over recent years, the media in the United Kingdom have been reflecting a concern about lone mothers that amounts to a moral panic. Even the broadsheet newspapers have articles like 'Alarm over teenage baby boom' (*Sunday Times*, 8 January 1992), which seems to assume that all teenage mothers are schoolgirls and unmarried. The BBC's *Panorama* programme 'Babies on Benefit' (1994) abandoned all but a thin veneer of balanced broadcasting to jump on the bandwagon of stigmatizing lone mothers as benefit scroungers.

Respected academics like Norman Dennis and A.H. Halsey (Dennis and Erdos 1992) have lent the weight of apparent sociological evidence in support of the belief that the children of lone parents do less well in life and cause more trouble than those brought up by their two biological parents. While these British 'communitarian' sociologists have not given such a reasoned and systematic analysis as their American counterparts (Wilson 1993; Etzioni 1994), neither have they gone as far in their policy recommendations as Charles Murray, who sees illegitimacy as 'the single most important social problem of our time' (Murray 1993) and withdrawing welfare benefits as the only way to re-establish the traditional norms of married parenthood. These academics on both sides of the Atlantic can be accused of 'feigning iconoclastic courage' (Stacey 1994: 56). They may indeed be a minority among sociologists, yet they have managed to win the ears of the political establishment as well as join in the populist chorus that derides their fellow sociologists as out-of-touch do-gooders. Apparently, 'even President Clinton is on the record as saying that Murray's analysis is essentially correct – though he said his solution was immoral' (Bunting 1994). At the Conservative Party Conference in 1993, the Home Secretary Michael Howard had words of praise for a scheme in New Jersey to remove welfare benefits from lone mothers who have a second or third child and the Housing Minister, Sir George Young, said that single parents under 21 had no right to local authority housing as their parents should be responsible for them.

All this concern is bad news for lone parents of all sorts. They are in fact a fairly heterogeneous bunch of people. Most of them (60 per cent) have become lone parents as a result of divorce or separation. Thirty per cent of all new babies are born outside marriage, 'illegitimate' children of formally 'single' mothers; but three quarters of these have their birth registered by two parents, mostly both living at the same address. And 16- to 19-year-olds constitute only 3 per cent of lone parents. Nevertheless, any smears about any sub-group of lone parents can get thrown into the pot and stirred up into a toxic brew to be administered to all of them.

In Britain, the process of stigmatization has been diverted somewhat by the row over the Child Support Act, 1991, which set up the Child Support Agency to pursue 'absent' parents for maintenance payments. A vociferous and effective lobby of separated fathers and their second families distracted attention away from the lone mothers themselves and succeeded in painting these men, who are in fact but the other half of the lone-parenting picture, in rather glowing colours. To some extent, this row has normalized lone parenthood and brought public consciousness into line with contemporary social realities. In fact, 18 per cent of women are now divorced by the age of 33 and as many as 24 per cent have been lone parents for some period before they reach that age, overwhelmingly because of marital breakdown (*Guardian*, report on National Child Development Study, 31 September 1993). Single mothers are not a deviant minority who can be readily marginalized, though they are – on average – an economically disadvantaged minority.

One of the most fascinating things about the attempt to demonize lone mothers is the assumptions it reveals about married motherhood and the family. In 1982 Michèle Barrett and I published a book called *The Anti-social Family*, in which we presented a socialist and feminist critique of the family. One of the things we argued was that 'the family' is as much a collective fantasy as a concrete institution, yet that the privileged place this fantasy gives to familial relations and the way in which other ties of intimacy and support are devalued and undermined mean that it has very real – and very negative – social effects. Kate Ellis (1981: 17) has described 'the family' as 'a metaphor for some private and public paradise lost'. Margaret Thatcher's 'return to Victorian values' and John Major's more mundane 'back to basics' are ways of expressing this backward-looking dream of a family that could meet all our personal needs and secure social harmony and national well-being at the same time. The current anxiety about lone motherhood is another expression of the same dream, and the social pathology of the lone mother is just as imaginary as the social desirability of the nuclear family.

Like all dreams, this one is full of jumps and narrative inconsistencies. At one moment, lone motherhood is presented as unnatural and married motherhood, by implication, as natural. The naturalizing of social phenomena is one of the commonest forms of ideological thought, here rendering monogamy as part of our human nature and adequately expressive of our natural psychological needs. At another moment, however, monogamy is seen as part of culture rather than nature. For Charles Murray, a central argument against lone mothers is that they cannot socialize the disruptive energy of their sons. Men are naturally unruly, but are civilized by their wives; only a father who is thus civilized can offer a suitable role model to his son (Bunting 1994).

Many of the negative stereotypes of lone parents have as their obverse the idealized images of married parenthood that feminists have exposed as dangerous fantasies. The idea of the lone mother as a benefit scrounger is the obverse of the married mother who turns happily and confidently to her husband for support. Feminists have pointed out that this economic dependence on an individual man has all sorts of negative consequences for women. It is associated with women's lack of power in family decision making, with an unequal division of labour in the home and with women's disadvantage in the labour market. What is more, women's dependence on a breadwinner who earns a real 'family wage', sufficient to support himself and his children, is to a large extent a myth (Barrett and McIntosh 1980). Among some groups in our society, particularly Afro-Caribbeans, such dependence has never been assumed. And even where it has been taken for granted, it has often been highly problematic; married women frequently have to look for paid work, not simply to supplement a shared 'family wage' but also to make sure that they have some income that is under their own control. If they are unable to find paid work, or cannot fit it in with their family responsibilities, they are thrown back onto a personal dependence that is often corrosive of spirit and self-esteem.

So critics who bewail the 'culture of dependency' among lone mothers should equally deplore family dependency. Some feminists have argued for the right of all non-employed people to some sort of independent income support benefit, regardless of whether they are married, cohabiting, living with other people or alone (London Women's Liberation Campaign 1979). Others have campaigned for family allowances: that society should offer 'direct financial provision for the maintenance of children', as Eleanor Rathbone (1940: ix) put it. Either of these would go some way towards tackling the real problem of mothers' dependence, which is dependence within marriage.

Giving the pejorative label 'dependency' to the claiming of state benefits is part of the whole pattern of the Conservative government's social thinking. The idea is that individuals and families should take care of themselves much more and not turn to the state for support. Lone parents show up all too starkly the fact that this is simply not possible for everyone. Either it is being assumed that those living with their children ought to go out to work to support the family, which goes against the idea that small children need a parent at home. Or it is assumed that somehow 'the family' will provide support, as if 'the family' could operate as a kind of private welfare system throughout society. Yet lone parents often do not have an 'absent parent', or any other relatives they can turn to, and many 'absent parents' have too many people who are supposed to be able to depend upon them.

It is true that lone mothers are more often in poverty than others. The 1992 General Household Survey found that 42 per cent of them had a gross weekly income of less than £100 and the percentage was even higher for those who had never been married. This greater poverty is associated with the fact that in Britain they are less likely to be in paid work: only 22 per cent of lone mothers with a child under 5 had a job and only 8 per cent a full-time job, compared with 47 per cent and 13 per cent for married or cohabiting mothers.

The image of absent fathers may have been rehabilitated to some extent by campaigns against the Child Support Agency, but they can still be presented as irresponsible and feckless. The assumed obverse image is the 'family man' who is responsible and respected, which again is a long way from the truth in many cases. Husbands do not always share their income with their families; many wives have to manage on inadequate housekeeping money and some even feel better off when they leave home and go onto state benefits than they did when they were relying on their husband for support. There are structural factors at work as well: as the costs of raising children increase, the number of men with steady and predictable incomes from secure 'permanent' employment decreases, so women can no longer feel confident that their husband will be able to support them. In addition, of course, many men are unemployed or disabled and are not able to maintain their families. When they claim benefit for the whole household, it may appear that they are supporting them, but in fact their wives and children are no less dependent on the state than lone-parent families.

Perhaps the most serious charge against lone parents is that they are ineffective at bringing up children. A.H. Halsey gives academic credence to this popular prejudice when he writes of children brought up by parents 'who do not follow the traditional norms', such as lone parents:

> On the evidence available, such children tend to die earlier, to have more illness, to do less well at school, to exist at a lower level of nutrition, comfort and conviviality, to suffer more unemployment, to be more prone to deviance and crime and, finally, to repeat the cycle of unstable parenting from which they themselves have suffered.
>
> (Dennis and Erdos 1992: xii)

The 'evidence' that such statements rely on relates to illegitimate children rather than to children of lone parents in general. It is also nearly twenty years old, coming from a period when lone parent-hood was rarer and more stigmatized than it is now. More careful studies suggest that it is hard to prove any detrimental effects because we do not know what group these children should be compared with. For instance, if you set out to discover the impact of divorce on children, you should not compare them with all children of intact marriages but with children of unhappily married parents who have decided not to divorce (Furstenberg and Cherlin 1991). Only then can you learn anything that could guide social policy on whether divorce should be easier or harder to obtain, or that could guide parents who want to break up. Judith Stacey (1994: 59) sums up the evidence very differently from Halsey: 'Research indicates that high-conflict marriages harm children more than do low-conflict divorces.' She goes on to say:

> In fact most children from both [two-parent and lone-parent] families turn out reasonably all right and when other parental resources – like income, education, self-esteem and a supportive

social environment – are roughly similar, signs of two-parent privilege largely disappear.

(Stacey 1994: 60)

Louie Burghes, Chapter 9 in this volume, also discusses the current debates about the disruption that lone parenting causes for children. She argues, on lines similar to Stacey's, that there is no evidence that children raised by a lone parent fare less well because these arguments are based on comparisons that are unreliable and biased against lone parenting. The problem is that the most disadvantaged one-parent children are being compared with the particularly well placed among those with two parents. Instead of exploring the reasons why they have problems, it is assumed that it is simply because they have only one parent and that the answer is to change the moral climate or the financial choices so that their parents are forced into marrying or staying married.

Married parenthood is far from being an ideal way of life. It is evidently a bad experience for the many parents who eventually divorce, but there is also a great deal of hidden ongoing disharmony, as we know from victim-report studies of marital rape, incest and violence between husband and wife, parents and children. This is particularly significant from a feminist point of view, as men are most often the perpetrators and women and girls the victims in these situations. Many relationships that do not have these frank forms of violence and abuse may be deeply unrewarding and lack any real intimacy or communication. The fact that a whole industry of family therapy has developed in recent years is testimony to the unsatisfactoriness of many family lives.

Within marriage, as well as outside it, women carry most of the responsibility for caring for children as well as any others who need looking after. The lack of child-care provision and state policies of 'community care' make this a heavy burden, especially in a period when our expectations for the quality of care, for both children and adults, are rising. Within marriage, much of this work goes unrecognized and unrewarded, and has to be combined with caring for the husband and playing the role of wife. Many women find that being on their own, without a husband, makes this work less burdensome. They can organize things as they wish and do not have to keep the children out of their father's hair or keep an old man from getting on his nerves.

It is not surprising, perhaps, that some of the images of lone motherhood reveal a deep ambivalence about marriage. The single mother is free and irresponsible, sexually promiscuous and available to men. By implication, the married mother is trapped and tied down and her sexuality controlled by her husband. Those who want to reverse what they see as the rising tide of lone motherhood often recognize that the only way to do this is through some form of coercion. The 'soft' methods would be increasing stigma and making divorce more difficult, which while not preventing separation might make it a harder choice to make. The 'hard' method is the financial one of cutting lone parents' rights to social security and tax breaks. As Judith Stacey puts it, 'historically, stable marriage systems rest on coercion, overt or veiled, and on inequality' (Stacey 1994: 65).

But why is it *women*'s ability to survive outside marriage – albeit often by the skin of their teeth – that has led to a rise in lone motherhood? Part of the answer must lie in the fact that marriage is more disadvantageous to women than to men. When women are less constrained to marriage, they more often prefer to avoid it. So the greater freedom of the lone woman highlights the lack of freedom of the married one.

Many of the discussions of lone motherhood are concerned with a comparison between lone mothers and an imaginary ideal of the married mother or with the ineffectiveness of lone parenting compared with a supposed model of dual parenting. But there is another dimension to the current anxiety, which is the notion that lone motherhood and irresponsible fatherhood are part of a self-reproducing underclass. The main element of continuity, it seems, in the new 'dangerous classes' is not criminality and moral degeneracy, as in the nineteenth century, but the culture of dependency and ineffective socialization.

The other side of this is the role that the family plays in the reproduction of all the social classes in society. In *The Anti-social Family*, Michèle Barrett and I argued that the reproduction of classes through family is a more significant social fact than intergenerational social mobility. Indeed, social mobility between generations is only worth talking about because there is an assumption that children will normally follow their parents and that higher-class fathers will be able to give their children more advantages than lower-class ones can. What we suggested was that the inheritance of wealth and the family support that helps children succeed in education are processes by which the family serves to reproduce the middle class. Many commentators see the same facts as evidence of the importance and value of the traditional family, since those children would not have done so well without it. But if we consider the family as a system throughout society, it becomes clear that it equally serves to reproduce the working class, where parents have no wealth to pass on and cannot give much backup to the children's schooling. So it is equally true to say that the children of unskilled workers would not have done so badly without the family. Overall, the family as an institution is essential to forming class divisions and handing them down from generation to generation.

One of the things that a consideration of lone parents shows up in a stark light is the paradox of this macro-sociological view of the family. For if it is really true that lone parents are reproducing an underclass, stuck in a pit below even the lower working class, then it becomes understandable that people in the higher classes value their family life, are grateful to their parents and see the family as a 'haven in a heartless world' (Lasch 1977) and a bastion against a predatory state and economic system. The same paradox can be found in racial divisions: they would not continue from generation to generation if it were not for the institution of the family which passes on racial identities; yet the subordinated racial groups urgently need their families to sustain a culture of resistance to racial indignity and a practical network of mutual support.

The family is fundamentally a selfish institution, encouraging a morality of 'charity begins at home', which is the antithesis of collectivist or truly communitarian values. It not only reproduces advantage and disadvantage, but it even more seriously disadvantages those who have small or weak families. So if lone mothers are stretched and disadvantaged it is because the family is such a privileged site of caring and mutual aid. It not only makes the rest of society *seem* bleak and unwelcoming, it also weakens non-familial networks and institutions that might provide support and comfort. In *The Anti-social Family* we concluded that 'caring, sharing and loving would be more widespread if the family did not claim them for its own' (Barrett and McIntosh 1982: 80).

So we were not only pointing to the 'dark' side of the family, as many critics have done, we were also seeking to understand what is appealing about family life. The paradox is that both exist side by side. Some people have good experiences, some have bad experiences, but the overall effect of the institutional dominance of the privatized family is to weaken community ties.

This paradox must be reflected in feminist campaigns as well. Though it is important to demonstrate that lone mothers do a good job and manage to be effective parents under adverse circumstances, it is also important to argue this in a way that does not assume an implicit approval of the conventional two-parent family. The point is not that one parent is as good as two, but that there are many problems about marriage and dual parenting that are highlighted by the rise in lone parenting (Millar 1994b). At the level of individuals, we need to ask: Why are couples breaking up so much? Why are some young mothers reluctant to marry at all? Why are women, rather than men, taking so much responsibility for children? And at the level of society: Why are there no perceived alternative forms of household or support network?

# Chapter 9

# Debates on disruption
## What happens to the children of lone parents[1]

*Louie Burghes*

It is tempting to say that society is and has long been concerned about the well-being of children who experience family disruption, or grow up in a lone parent family, or both. While historically many children lost a parent through death, it is parental separation (of married or cohabiting couples) and divorce that characterize most family disruption today.

It is about the consequences for children who have witnessed the breakup of their family in this way that much of the relatively recent anxiety has been concerned and from which much of the original research in the field has stemmed. In Britain, both were reactions to a divorce rate that began to rise in the 1960s and had increased sixfold by the 1980s. In 1992, almost fourteen in every thousand married persons obtained a divorce (Office of Population Censuses and Surveys 1994). At current rates, almost four in ten of today's marriages will end in divorce (Haskey 1993).

It is perhaps not surprising that the more than doubling in the number of lone-parent families in Britain in the past twenty years – to more than 1¼ million lone parents with 2¼ million dependent children (Haskey 1994) – again kindled public debate at the beginning of the 1990s. The well-being of their children has not been, however, the only concern, and the recent and vehement attacks on lone parents, and particularly never-married lone mothers, may have other or additional causes and reflect different concerns (*The Times* 1991; McGlone 1994). At least two may be discerned. The first is the rising social security cost associated with increasing family breakdown and lone parenthood (Department of Social Security 1993a). The second is anxiety that the increase in single (never-married) lone motherhood reflects a demise of the 'traditional', intact two-parent family. For some social and political commentators, this represents the loss of a central building block of society, and a 'coherent' if non-Utopian strategy for the socialization and rearing of the next generation (Halsey 1991; Dennis and Erdos 1992). In looking, therefore, at what happens to children who experience family disruption or lone parenthood or both compared with those who do not, there is concern about the well-being of the children, but there is also anxiety about the consequences for society. These two very different interests may be thought to reflect, perhaps rather arbitrarily, how children fare compared to how they behave and how society fares.

Some aspects of the physical, psychological, social and economic development, behaviour and achievement of children who have experienced family disruption, lone parenthood or both have been explored in research. Some aspects of their development have been tracked through their teens and into early adulthood. The employment, unemployment, occupational status and income of young people and young adults have also been investigated, as have their transitions to adulthood (leaving school and starting work, for example) and family formation. These various aspects of their development are referred to here as the 'outcomes'. The issues of delinquency and criminal behaviour and their possible causes tend to have been researched separately from these developmental enquiries (Utting *et al.* 1993). The findings are reported briefly here.

There are five further sections to this chapter. The first considers the development of research into 'outcomes' for children in the light of family formation and family change. The second addresses the issue of 'how good are the data' with which these outcomes are measured and on which judgements are made. The third section looks at what the research findings tell us about family disruption, lone parenthood and the outcomes for children and young people, and the fourth considers what might account for these findings. The chapter ends by considering what might underlie the different ways in which children respond to family disruption and its aftermaths and what and how these might provide lessons for the positive benefit of families and children.

## FAMILY CHANGE AND DEVELOPMENTS IN RESEARCH ON OUTCOMES

The way in which the concern for children and their outcomes is often expressed in public debate is in terms specifically of their being the children of lone parents. Similarly, their experience of this family life in a lone-parent family is implicitly characterized by two facts: first, that all lone-parent families and all experiences of family change and disruption are the same; second, that this is a static model along the lines of 'once a lone-parent family always a lone-parent family'. But research has had to take into account that neither of these are the case. Lone-parent families comprise not only those that come about because of separation or divorce, but also (although less frequently) those resulting from bereavement or (and more commonly now than was once the case) those who are single and have never been married. The picture is further complicated by cohabitation and re-partnership. Among the latter, moreover, there is a considerable diversity of family structure and family life (Robinson and Smith 1993).

In 1992, almost 170,000 children under 16 years old in Britain experienced the divorce of their parents (OPCS 1994) and almost one in four children are likely to do so before they reach 16 (Haskey 1990). Provisional estimates suggest that there were nearly 750,000 separated or divorced lone mothers in 1992 with on average almost two dependent children (Haskey 1994). There are as well those children who have experienced the breakdown of their parents' cohabiting partnership. There are no official statistics on how many children are affected in this way and the lone-mother families created as a result are recorded as single (never-married) lone mothers (Brown 1995). There are still those (even if their numbers are smaller now than they once were) who experience the death of a parent. The most recent count, for 1992, provisionally estimated that there were 60,000 widows heading lone-parent families with on average less than two children per family (Haskey 1994). Also growing numbers of children are living with their never-married lone mother and no resident partner. They may have done so from birth or since the breakdown in her cohabiting relationship. The number of single lone-mother families was estimated provisionally to be 490,000 at the last count, in 1992. They have the smallest average family size at 1.4 dependent children (Haskey 1994).

The number of lone-father families has also grown in recent years, even though they account for a declining proportion of the total number of lone parents. A provisional estimate, again for 1992, puts their number at 120,000.

Lone parenthood, however, is no more a static state than are other family forms. Just as lone-parent families are formed, so they may dissolve through re-partnerships whether of cohabitation or marriage (as well as through the death of a parent or when a young person grows up). Periods of lone parenthood are commonly around four years (Mckay and Marsh 1994).

The combined result of these family changes is that more children, though still a minority, experience more family change and experience life in a diversity of families and family structures. Second or step-families may comprise, for example, combinations of 'his', 'her' and 'their' children. How children respond to these changes will not be uniform and the nature of the experience and their response to it cannot be assumed. Their relationships with their own parents, for example, may get better or worse; they may see more of them or less – not that frequency and quality of contact should necessarily be assumed synonymous. Indeed, the qualitative elements of the child–parent relationships are likely to be critical influences on their well-being and development. In addition, children may gain and lose siblings – stepbrothers and stepsisters and/or half brothers and half sisters. While some grandparents, aunts and uncles may become more distant, others may become closer and new ones appear.

Change and diversity may seem to be the hallmarks of family life for increasing numbers of children today as more of them experience the breakdown of their parents' relationship, family life with one resident and one non-resident parent and/or the formation of a second family. It may be important, therefore, to remember the context of family life within which most children are brought up in Great Britain. Indeed, given the emphasis on the rapidity and diversity of family change, it may come as some surprise that seven out of ten dependent children live with both their natural parents (International Year of the Family 1994). This compares with two in ten children living with a lone parent and one in ten in a step-family. Despite their common family structure, however, children's experience of life in an 'intact' family and of growing up should not be assumed to be uniform. Once again, within any family structure, family life will be played out with great diversity and variety.

As already indicated, research initially tended to concentrate on children whose parents had separated or divorced. This was not surprising given anxiety about the increasing prevalence of divorce from the 1960s. The focus of concern, moreover, was the divorce itself, the consequences of which were thought of as a relatively short-term crisis. As divorce became more widespread, the debate about its consequences broadened. Family life both before and after the divorce were also considered, even if the divorce itself remained in many respects the focal point. Divorce thus began to be seen as part of a process of family change. It might be preceded by marital disharmony, conflict and even violence and result in lone parenthood and perhaps the establishment of a second family. Research thus began to address the possibility of influences on children's well-being and outcomes over a longer period, and of longer-term consequences for children both in second families and in their subsequent transitions into (more independent) adulthood.

The consequences of these experiences of family change for children, and their development as young people and into adulthood, are usually compared and contrasted with those of children in both intact and bereaved families. What research has not done (and perhaps given their limited number in longitudinal cohorts, could not have done) is an equivalent assessment for the (now growing number of) children of single (never-married) lone mothers. Some of these children will always have lived on their own with their mothers. The experience of others, whose parents had a cohabiting relationship but are now separated, is assumed to have been more akin to children whose married parents have separated or divorced. It is interesting to reflect, perhaps, that those children born to a single mother who subsequently but not initially cohabits with the child's father will experience family change to become part of a 'traditional' two-parent family.

Commonly measured outcomes include academic achievement – as measured by reading and arithmetic tests (at 7, 11 and 16 years in the National Child Development Study) – and educational qualifications and psychological adjustment and behaviour.

## HOW GOOD ARE THE DATA?

It is often easier in social enquiries to pose concerns and ask questions than to answer them. To what extent can the data available be taken as telling us definitively and with surety about the relationship between children's experience of family life and family change and their well-being and achievement in childhood and adulthood and over a wide range of social, educational and economic indicators?

Researchers do, in fact, encounter a number of methodological problems and may advise care and caution in the interpretation of the results. A number of these arise because, despite the interest in and concern about children and the effect on children of family structure and family change, little research has been designed specifically to consider the effects on them in the long term. Researchers have had more frequently to use data collected as by-products of other work or in research designed for other purposes.

A common critique of clinical studies, for example, has been that the sample from which the data are drawn is not representative of all children facing family disruption and the findings, therefore, cannot be taken as applying to them all, nor are they suitable for drawing conclusions about the children's development over time. Moreover, without a control group of children who have neither lived in a lone-parent family nor experienced family disruption, there is no benchmark against which to measure whether and by how much the outcomes of the one group differ from that of the other.

National representative longitudinal cohort studies offer solutions to some of these problems. Such surveys do, for example, enable the outcomes for children with different experiences of family structure and change to be compared. Similarly, where data are available for the same children at different points in their childhood as well as in their adolescence and adulthood, it is possible to see whether any observed differences between their outcomes and those of their peers in intact families change over time and to allow for the possibility of these to be short or long term. This is important because problems may abate. Stress and strain may ease, for example, and behaviour and psychological difficulties improve. The 'effects' may wash out with time; children may 'catch up' lost ground in their educational achievement, for example. On the other hand, problems suppressed in childhood at the time of the disruption and in its aftermath may emerge later, perhaps as difficulties in their own relationships.

Such studies are not, however, without their own limitations, including their limited number. While the three major national longitudinal studies available to researchers were all designed to look at various aspects of children's development and achievement – whether physical, psychological, social and/or economic – they were not selected or designed specifically to measure the effects of family disruption and lone parenthood.[2] What measures of development and achievement are available from these studies may not be suitable or ideal to assess the effects, if any and in whatever direction, on children from their experiences of family disruption and lone parenthood. For example, are the measures of achievement in mathematics and reading at various stages in children's education career, which the surveys do provide, more valuable and relevant than measures of quick or logical thinking, earlier maturity or a more flexible approach to life? Again, some forms of antisocial behaviour that are measured might be balanced by other positive behaviour that is not.

The data available also need to be interpreted with care. There may be more than one interpretation of behaviour instinctively thought of as a 'good' or 'bad' outcome. Too much quiet and compliant behaviour may indicate suppressed emotions, which may be damaging to young people's relationships in the long run rather than reflecting psychological adjustment and well-being. Similarly, the disruptive behaviour said to be characteristic of boys in reaction to the stress and upheaval of family disruption may be more psychologically protective in the long run (Chase-Lansdale and Hetherington 1990).

These findings, moreover, are average outcomes for groups of children. They ought not to be taken, but sometimes are, as being applicable to individual children. As averages they disguise 'better' and 'worse' outcomes achieved by all children, whatever their family experience.

Nor is the observation of a statistically significant association – between some measured outcome and family disruption – a guarantee that a causal relationship exists. Researchers are clearly well aware of this and try to take account of other causal influences. But it is not yet guaranteed that they have always done so. We cannot be certain, for example, that all possible factors (other than marital disruption and lone parenthood) that may account for the observed relationship have been fully taken into account. There may be intervening variables that account for the observed association, the control variables themselves may be inadequately measured or the direction of the causal relationship may be other than is generally supposed. Financial hardship and poverty, for example, may be a cause or an effect of family change or both. Social class, income, children's age and gender are all obvious factors that may be influential. While they need to be taken into account, researchers have not or are not always able to do so or to do so satisfactorily. Nor are these the only factors that may be important in determining how children fare, yet few others have been taken directly into account. It has been suggested, for example, that a causal relationship may not hold when other influential factors, such as marital conflict and parents' ages at the time of the child's birth, are taken into account and that the findings presented in the next section may be shown not to hold when investigated further (Kiernan 1992a; Ní Bhrolcháin 1992; Burghes 1994). Comparison should be made of the effects on children of family disruption and lone parenthood with the effects on children of other social and economic influences, such as parental unemployment, and their own poor health or inadequate education.

The way in which the outcomes are themselves defined and measured may be questioned, as may the statistical techniques applied to them and the interpretation of the results (Ní Bhrolcháin 1992, 1993). Moreover, while longitudinal data have their advantages, the large time differences between the events and the measured outcomes lead to wariness about concluding that there are causal relationships. By the time the children of divorced parents reach adulthood, for example, the experience of their parents' divorce may have been many years earlier, and there may have been many intervening experiences that will have influenced their 'outcomes'.

There is also the difficulty of ensuring that measurements of children's development are identical at different points in time. Can we be sure that a test of arithmetic at 16 years is equivalent to and as appropriate as that used to measure their attainment at 7 years? And can we know what sorts of measure of behaviour and psychological well-being would be thought equivalent at the two ages? Even if these difficulties are resolved, there remains the issue of what magnitude of difference – between the outcomes of children from different family settings and with different experiences of family life – would be thought to be significant to warrant concern or a social policy response?

That much of the research in this field has had to rely on two of the three longitudinal data sets (see note 2) raises the issue of how, or in what way, results from these studies of children born in the mid-1940s and late 1950s can be considered applicable to children experiencing family disruption or lone parenthood today. Not only is family life today structured very differently from how it was then, but more families have experienced family disruption, and more children their parents' parting and living apart. This may have changed both the baseline measurement of outcomes for children in intact families and the outcomes for the children experiencing such disruption. Whether children's outcomes will be different as a result of their experiences being more normative will in part depend on how the experiences of family disruption and life as part of a lone-parent family themselves affect the development of children. If social stigma is a major player it might be expected that there would have been some amelioration over time in its effects. On the other hand, if individual and family relations at a personal level are more predominant influences, the effects may have changed little as a result of the their greater prominence. In all likelihood, however, both social stigma and personal relations are influential.

Looking to the United States, with its longer history both of divorce and of research into its consequences, researchers were first of the somewhat gloomy opinion that there seemed to have been little ameliorating effect on outcomes from divorce being more wide-spread. There are, however, some suggestions now that the conse-quences of divorce are less severe than was previously the case.[3] Better welfare provision and the prevailing attitude towards divorce are thought to account for the relatively less damaging effects of parental divorce on children in Scandinavia than in Britain. As Martin Richards (1994) cautions, however, data are not available to test these ideas satisfactorily.

## FINDINGS FROM THE RESEARCH[4]

A short-hand summary of the research findings suggests that, on the one hand, nothing can with certainty be said about how any child will develop merely from knowing that he or she comes from a lone-parent family or a two-parent family – second or intact. On the other hand, if the data are reliable, on average, the prospects for children who have experienced particular types of family disruption or single lone parenthood are lower over a range of outcomes than they are for those living continuously with both their parents. The differences may be relatively small, but researchers report a consistent pattern of such findings from a number of studies of similar issues. Neither family disruption nor family structure *per se*, however, seems alone to account for these disparities, but rather the *type* of disruption experienced. Children from widowed lone-parent families, for exam-ple, often do not fare markedly worse than their peers in intact families.

These 'better' outcomes are often contrasted with the 'poorer' average outcomes of children who have experienced lone parenthood as a result of marital breakdown (i.e. the separation or divorce of their parents) compared with children in intact families. These 'poorer' average outcomes for children are not solely a consequence of the divorce; some, and sometimes much, of the measured effects – in behaviour and educational attainment – have been found to occur *beforehand*. The observed differences in outcomes may then continue after the divorce but not necessarily worsen. This may suggest that divorce as an event does not measure the beginning of the breakdown in the marital relationship or its quality and influence on children's development. Rather, it is the quality of the family relationships, of which the divorce is only a part, that are influential.

Research also suggests that differences can be observed between those who have and have not experienced particular types of family disruption on outcomes not measurable until adulthood. Among those considered are employment, unemployment, occupational status and income as well as health and social behaviour. It is not possible in a brief review to do justice to the complexity of the research or the subtle variations in outcome findings.

In general, once account is taken of other possible influential factors, social class being the most obvious example, the gap in outcomes between children who have and have not experienced family change narrows. In some cases they disappear; in others, statistically significant differences may remain. Some of these differences are small. A number of researchers have reported such or a similar pattern of findings.

Just three examples of the research findings are presented here. The first looks at the behaviour and psychological adjustment of children who have and have not experienced family disruption and lone parenthood; the second looks at educational qualifications and labour market attachment in adulthood. The comparative experiences of their transitions to adulthood are also considered.

Elsa Ferri (1976) examined the home and school behaviour of children at 11 years in one- and two-parent families. Account was taken of the cause of the lone parenthood. At *school*, the behaviour of children whose parents had divorced was rated as poorer and they were considered to be less well adjusted than children living either with both their biological parents or with a widowed mother. However, the statistical significance of the findings disappeared when other factors were allowed for and low income was a particularly important factor in this respect.[5] Of course, for many lone-parent families, their low income may be the result of their family disruption.

Ferri's work is alone in taking family income so directly into account in this way as far as outcomes for children are concerned.[6] Direct measures such as she used are rarely available and proxies, such as social class, are often inadequate (Burghes 1994).

Ferri's findings showed little statistically significant variation in the rating of the behaviour of children from different family settings by their *parents*. This was particularly relevant for those from intact and widowed lone-mother families. However, divorced and separated mothers were more likely to report that their children, particularly the girls, were having difficulties or displaying disturbed behaviour. These findings, as Ferri points out, are based on the parents' perceptions of their children's behaviour, which may have been influenced by their family circumstances and changes to it. Family disruption might have made them more conscious of their children's behaviour and anxious about its cause (Ferri 1976).

Jane Elliott and Martin Richards (1991) and Andy Cherlin *et al.* (1991) took the analysis of children's behaviour one stage further. Both studies looked at children and young people's behaviour both before and after the divorce of their parents, as well as in comparison with children in intact families. All but one of the results found that while children who had experienced the separation or divorce of their parents displayed 'poorer' behaviour than those who did not, it was no worse after the divorce than beforehand.[7]

Research assessments of the educational qualifications of young people and young adults suggest that outcomes are influenced by the nature of the marital disruption. This pattern is repeated in employment, unemployment and occupational status (Maclean and Wadsworth 1988; Kuh and Maclean 1990; Elliott and Richards 1991; Richards and Elliott n.d.). In each case – whether it is their chances of getting educational qualifications, being in employment rather than unemployed or the level of their income and their occupational status, and after controlling for social class or level of mother's education – the outcomes for the young people and young adults' outcomes were lower for those who had experienced the separation and divorce of their parents than for those whose parents had remained together. Richards and Elliott (n.d.) observed that for young people with fathers in non-manual occupations who had experienced the separation or divorce of their parents, the chances of achieving any educational qualifications were reduced and were akin to those with fathers in manual occupations whose parents stayed together.

In general, the outcomes for those who have experienced bereavement are little if at all different from those who have not done so. Subsequent research on further family change has shown that the effects on children of becoming part of a second family also seem to vary according to the type of disruption preceding it. New relationships following bereavement are associated with as good (occasionally better) average outcomes compared with children living with both their natural parents. Yet the comparison is often unfavourable between children whose parent lives with a new partner following separation or divorce and their peers from intact families (Kiernan 1992b; Cockett and Tripp 1994).

A further line of enquiry has compared the 'transitions to adulthood' made by young people. These 'transitions' include age of leaving education (and whether this was for financial reasons), of entering full-time employment, of leaving home (and whether for 'negative' reasons[8]), of cohabiting or getting married and of becoming a parent. Kathleen Kiernan (1992b) found that, overall, where family change or disruption was due to marital breakdown this was associated with young people making earlier adult transitions compared with children from intact families and that the differences were statistically significant. Little or no difference in the age of transition was found when comparing young people who lost a parent through death and whose parents had remained together. This general finding held whether their remaining parent had re-partnered or remarried or not. Kiernan (1992b) observed that the cause of the disruption rather than the disruption *per se* seemed important in affecting these transitions. None the less, the cause of the disruption seemed to be more important and influential for boys than for girls and the disruption itself more influential for girls.

Similar 'transition to adulthood' outcomes were analysed by Ní Bhrolcháin (1993). She concludes that the data do not allow the results to be considered as more than provisional, nor do they 'suggest that the group differences observed [here] *result from* the family experiences of the children involved' (Ní Bhrolcháin 1994: 24). She comments as well that, while the data suggest some association between the two (the observed outcomes and the family experience), 'the children of disrupted families are not distinctive in their experience' (p. 25). While most children from all family groups leave school at the minimum school leaving age, none of the other outcomes is 'the norm' for children who have experienced family disruption.

Given the hue and cry about never-married lone mothers – and a debate that implies a degree of certainty about the development of their children – it may come as some surprise that there has been very little comparable research about either the development of their children or their experience of family life. There were very few such children in the longitudinal surveys of the 1940s and 1950s (where they were defined as 'illegitimate') and findings for them have been analysed only up to the age of 11 years. In general, their average life chances were found to be lower at birth compared with children from two-parent intact families, although their subsequent physical development was adequate. Measures of academic achievement suggested that these were likely to be lower for children of single lone parents than for those in intact two-parent families. But their results are not necessarily as low as those of children from a manual occupation family background whose parents have separated or divorced (Ferri 1976). Better results had been found on some measures by illegitimate children who remained living with their mother alone than by those who subsequently lived with both of their parents. This might suggest (as is discussed later) that it is the changes in relationships that such transitions bring rather than the family setting *per se* that are influential. The sample base for these findings was, however, very small.

The rise in the divorce rate since the 1960s has been linked in the public mind with apparently increasing criminal and delinquent behaviour of young people – or more accurately that of boys and young men. Research has found that children from backgrounds of multiple deprivation are more likely to engage in delinquent behaviour and that the same is true for children who have experienced the separation or divorce of their parents – but with a weight towards minor offences (Utting *et al.* 1993). However, it is also the case that neither family disruption nor deprivation *per se* alone accounts for this. Rather it is, in aspects of children's upbringing, particularly the nature and consistency of the care provided by, and their relationship with, their parents that is most influential. In other words, 'The *direct* influence on children's behaviour is... seen to be the quality of the relationship with, and between, their parents' (Utting *et al.* 1993: 20).

David Farrington (1994) describes three aspects of parent care that may be influential in this way. These are discipline (which should not be excessively harsh or inconsistent), supervision (parents need to be watchful and monitor their children's activities) and parental attitude (warm and loving parents tend not to have delinquent children). Multiple deprivation and family disruption appear at first sight directly influential because they make it more difficult for parents to establish and maintain relationships and a home environment protective against delinquent behaviour. But they do not preclude it; indeed, there are circumstances in which the reverse may be the case.

## WHY POORER OUTCOMES?

Researchers have looked to a range of social, financial and psychological factors to account for differences in outcomes where they exist.

These factors may have preceded the disruption, occurred afterwards or both. They illuminate the reality and variation in the lives of children caught up in family change and disruption.

On the psychological dimension, family disruption, with or without conflict, is likely to be stressful and upsetting. Children are frequently reported to suffer from a loss of self-esteem. They may, although not inevitably, experience reduced or 'diminished' parenting and perhaps limited or lost contact with a parent. Domestic life may be more chaotic and less certain and secure. Supportive, attentive and authoritative parenting, which increases children's welfare, may be limited, in the short term at least, by parents' own distress.

Children may have experienced intense psychological stress and distress where family life has been characterized by disharmony, conflict or violence, particularly where they have witnessed or been embroiled in it. The more intense and long-lasting are the stress and distress, the greater are the behaviour and psychological consequences likely to be (Chase-Lansdale and Hetherington 1990). For these children their parents' parting may provide relief and allow them to establish or improve and enjoy relationships with each separately. On the other hand, some marriages and cohabiting relationships end without conflict. Moreover, disharmony between separating parents may increase as, for example, financial arrangements have to be made and visits between children and their now non-resident parent agreed (Cockett and Tripp 1994).

It is unlikely that all parental relationships are characterized by conflict before they break down, nor that the conflict is always witnessed by their children. The discovery by researchers, therefore, that children's outcomes may be affected even before their parents part suggests the possibility of more subtle links between the quality of family relationships and children's well-being and development.

Disrupted and lone-parent families frequently have diminished, inadequate and insecure incomes. Indeed recent research by Martin Richards and Jane Elliott (n.d.) has found that, on the point of separation, these families in all social groups were much more likely to be experiencing financial hardship than were those who remained together. Research has rarely been able to assess how much of any difference in outcome between children from lone and intact families might be accounted for by low family income *per se*.[9] Limited financial resources, and the extent to which family income is suddenly reduced, creates practical difficulties in caring adequately for children and adds stress. Impoverished living standards may well have adverse consequences for children, limiting, for example, their ability to achieve in school (Ferri 1976; McLanahan 1988). Some young people may leave school and/or home earlier than they would otherwise have done because of financial hardship.

Family disruption may mean having to move home and school; neither may be welcome or easy for children and both may entail the loss of supportive school, family and social networks and the security, familiarity and continuity that these provide in children's everyday lives.

## CHILDREN'S DEVELOPMENT COMPARED

Research into the outcomes for children who have or have not experienced family disruption and the accompanying debate is complex, contentious and controversial. On the one hand there are those wary of the quality of the data available and what can safely be said about children's outcomes as a result. On the other hand, there is the sense that outcomes must evidently be poorer for children who experience family disruption and lone parenthood (than for those who do not) because of their distress and frequently poorer socio-economic circumstances.

In between, a number of researchers feel confident about the poorer outcomes where they have been found for children and young people who have experienced family disruption, because of similar such findings from a number of studies (and cross-nationally). The differences between the outcomes, they acknowledge, may not be large and there is less certainty about accounting for them; the complex web of causation has yet to be untangled. Doing so is thought to be neither simple nor straightforward. Why, for example, are there children experiencing family disruption who fare 'well' and others in two-parent intact families who fare 'badly'? Neither experience of family life will be 'all good' or 'all bad'; such a model is too simplistic a view of the realities and dynamics of family life. Conflict and poor socio-economic circumstances, after all, may and do occur in two-parent families.

Where children who experience family disruption are likely to differ from those who do not is in facing more and more difficult circumstances, events and changes in their lives. But such an analysis also allows that the reverse will sometimes be the case, and that the breakup of a family may make relations more harmonious.

The fact that some children fare worse than others is likely to reflect

the interrelationship between the particular pathway of these circumstances, family events, the stage of development and maturity of the
children as they occur, as well as their relationship with their parents.
The relationship between their parents will have its effect too and
there is no given path that it will travel as families part.

It is possible, therefore, that the apparently poorer outcomes for
children from step-families, for example, may be due in part at least to
the greater number of such potentially difficult transitions that they
have to make (Capaldi and Patterson 1991; Capaldi 1992). For many
this will have been their second family change – for example, from
living with their own natural parents, to living with one parent alone,
and then to living with their own parent and a step-parent.

Such an interpretation is thought to be in keeping with stress
theories, which assume that the effects of family disruption arise from
the transitions and changes in relationships and not the family setting
*per se*, generally lone parenthood, that follows (McLanahan and
Bumpass 1988). For while it is possible that every transition might be
done carefully, none the less each might still be difficult and may
require psychological adjustments to new family relationships and
social circumstances. Clearly the relationships between individuals
within step-families are complex and the psychological adjustment
required greater (Robinson and Smith 1993). Moreover, just as new
relationships may be gained (as is often said about boys and
stepfathers), others may be 'lost' (as girls are said to feel sometimes
about their relationship with their mother).

Researchers seem increasingly of the view that there is no single
explanation, whether psychological, sociological or economic, for the
generally poorer outcomes that children who have experienced family
disruption may display compared with those from intact families.
There could be no single explanation that would fit the different
experiences of family change. But that is not to say that some sorts of
explanation might be more likely for some types of change or
disruption, or at different times or of different intensities. Some
researchers suggest the need for a multi-dimensional model based on
the concepts of 'resources', which provide opportunities to develop
social and cognitive competence to help deal with 'stressors', that is
stressful life events such as marital dissolution and the psychological,
social and economic difficulties that it entails (Amato 1993). Others
suggest, perhaps in similar vein, the need to consider not so much
whether a particular factor is present or absent, but the total
'configuration' of these resources and stressors. Not only, therefore,

might one resource compensate for the lack of another, but pre-divorce stressors could exceed those post-divorce (Demo 1993).

The discovery of pre-divorce effects on children's outcomes might add weight to the theory that the 'cause' of children's outcomes is the relationship between the dynamics of the marriage itself (in turn affected by partner pre-selection) and the (changing) social and economic circumstances and events that families experience. Divorce is just one social event (albeit an important one) within this process (Richards 1993).

It is perhaps important to reflect, however, that there will be children for whom the separation and divorce of their parents will not be a damaging long-term experience. Nor do we know whether children for whom it is a damaging experience would have been better off had their parents stayed together. We do not know what the outcomes for these children would have been had they done so. But nor can we be certain that where the relationship between their parents is marked by discord, children will always be better off if they part. To do so is to assume that such conflict would have continued. We do not know what will happen to either group of children in the future. We can never assume that families will stay as they are either in the nature of their relationships or in their structure.

## NOTES

1 This chapter is based on a project funded by the Joseph Rowntree Foundation. It reviewed British research on the comparative development and well-being of children who had and had not experienced family disruption, lone parenthood or both. A report, *Lone Parenthood and Family Disruption: The Outcomes for Children*, was published in 1994 by the Family Policy Studies Centre, London.
2 These studies are the 1970 British Cohort Study, the National Child Development Study (1958) and the National Survey of Health and Development (1946).
3 Personal communication with Martin Richards, Centre for Family Research, Cambridge University.
4 For a more detailed account of the research and a fuller report of the findings, see Burghes 1994.
5 These other factors were gender, social class (family income), family size, receipt of free school meals, access to basic household amenities, parental aspirations and employment situation and whether children were even in care.
6 Martin Richards (Centre for Family Research, University of Cambridge) has done so for outcomes in adulthood. This work is not yet published. See Burghes (1994).

7   The work by Andrew Cherlin and colleagues compared the outcomes for children in Britain and the United States. The exception to the general finding was for girls from lone-parent families in the United States, who displayed somewhat fewer behaviour problems than other American girls from intact families.
8   These 'negative' reasons might be, for example, friction between family members or poor home accommodation.
9   The work by Elsa Ferri (1976), already referred to, is an exception to this.

# Chapter 10

# Social constructions of lone motherhood

## A case of competing discourses

*Ann Phoenix*

Since the 1980s, the media in Britain and the United States have made many negative pronouncements on lone mothers. The notion of 'feckless mothers', who get pregnant in order to obtain welfare payments and housing and then rear children who are likely to become criminal, has been much aired by underclass theorists (such as Charles Murray 1990). Such notions have been picked up by politicians (including Bill Clinton as the Democratic president of the United States and Dan Quayle when he was the Republican vice-president) and by various British Conservative Secretaries of State. While many of these pronouncements have used moral arguments, of 'responsible parenting' and maintenance of 'traditional families', their proposed remedies to these 'problems' have been designed to reduce the economic dependence on the state of lone parents (who are predominantly lone mothers; Burghes 1993) and their children. They have produced a construction of lone mothers as 'feckless', wilfully responsible for the poverty that has been well documented to be a feature of lone parenting (Bradshaw and Millar 1991; Burghes 1993) and undeserving of either public sympathy or economic support.

A major aim of the legislation and proposals regarding lone mothers (in Britain and the USA) has been to save the treasury money. Thus, in Britain there have been several measures to enforce 'parental responsibility'. The most important are:

1  The setting up, in 1993, of the Child Support Agency (in operation of the 1991 Child Support Act) as an attempt to force errant fathers, rather than the welfare state, to be economically responsible for their children.
2  Holding parents responsible for their under-age children's crimes and hence any penalties enforced on children. There are also now

regulations compelling parents to make provision for any children that their children (of up to 17 years of age) have (McLagan 1992).
3  In London, Wandsworth Council's attempt to force lone mothers back to either their parents' or male partner's homes by offering them nothing other than temporary housing. This action was bolstered by legislation removing responsibility from local authorities for homeless people.

The assumption (by politicians and journalists) that there is still a popular consensus that lone mothers are problematic to the state, society and all 'decent' tax-payers has implications for the ways in which lone mothers are treated. If pervasive discourses on lone mothers construct them as problematic and irresponsible, then denouncements and financial penalties against those who are lone mothers are justified as necessary for the deterrence of others. Recent British discourses and policy share some similarities with those policies previously adopted in parts of the USA (Kahn and Kamerman 1988). There has also been some interest in Britain in the New Jersey (USA) policy of refusing Aid to Families with Dependent Children to those who have a second child while single and dependent on state provision.

Positive potential economic solutions, such as the provision of adequate and cheap child care so that lone mothers can take themselves out of the poverty trap through employment (Bradshaw and Millar 1991; Burghes 1993), have not been given the same consideration as punitive policies (see Millar, Chapter 5 in this volume, and Edwards and Duncan, Chapter 6; also Millar 1995).

Negative discourses of lone mothers are sufficiently pervasive to constitute a 'discursive formation' (Foucault 1972) where many pronouncements fit together to construct lone mothers as deviant and problematic. Popularized through the media, these constructions have taken on the appearance of objective reality, at least to some people. However, there have also been discursive constructions that have countered notions of lone motherhood as problematic and hence have prevented them from continuing to be widely accepted as 'regimes of truth' (Foucault 1980; Hall 1992).

The first part of this chapter examines the ways in which these competing discourses make lone motherhood a contested terrain. It argues that negative constructions do underpin relations of power between 'lone mothers' and others, but that there are other discourses that oppose such negative constructions and demonstrate that they do not provide a sound basis for the development of social policy.

The second part of the chapter considers the contradictions that have made discourses of 'race' silent in recent 'moral panics' about lone motherhood. Although there have been articles that have examined current popular discourses of 'father-absence' in the 'Afro-Caribbean community' (e.g. Alibhai-Brown 1994), 'race' has generally not featured in recent discourses on lone parents. This absence is notable because it is commonplace for writings that highlight 'the problems of black people', black people as problematic or black people in general to focus on the high percentages of black households that are lone-mother households (Younge 1995; Forna 1995). The Swann report on the 'educational underachievement' of black children largely blamed this on lone motherhood (Swann 1985). Lone motherhood and its concomitant 'father absence' has long been blamed for the 'criminality' of young men, particularly those who are black and/or working class (see the critique by Griffin 1993). While a confidential Cabinet office paper leaked to the *Guardian* in November 1993 stressed that there is no evidence to suggest that lone-parent families are 'criminogenic' (Hewitt and Leach 1993), notions that there are links between lone motherhood and children's delinquency are commonplace. It is thus not surprising, for example, that Charles Murray (the New Right ideologue who has done most to disseminate the 'underclass thesis' in Britain) has argued that black people are at the forefront of underclass trends (Abbott and Wallace 1992). This part of the chapter argues that, although the silence on black families in recent attacks on lone mothers may seem positive, it is not necessarily so.

## CHALLENGES TO DISCOURSES OF LONE MOTHERS

In July 1993, John Redwood, then Secretary of State for Wales, made a speech against lone mothers that set the tone for a major theme of the Conservative party annual conference at the beginning of October 1993. At that conference, various British Secretaries of State attacked lone motherhood in a way that echoed sentiments expressed in the US 1992 presidential campaign and that could be viewed as attempts to provide a context in which the new Child Support Agency could pursue 'errant fathers'. Michael Howard, the then Home Secretary, and Peter Lilley, the Social Security Secretary, both made speeches that questioned whether unmarried, single women should have children and, if they did, whether they should have access to council housing and welfare payments. They thus paved the way for the Green Paper on housing, which aimed to restrict the housing entitlement of lone mothers (announced by Sir George Young in 1993). John Patten, the then Secretary of State for Education, spoke of the hordes of irresponsible parents in Britain who have children and then fail to look after them properly, a sentiment that fitted with Michael Howard's claim at the conference that the children of lone mothers are likely to become criminals and his advocacy of a return to a policy of having the babies born to young, single women adopted: 'So the outcome was that girls in that situation frequently put their babies out for adoption as the only way out. From the child's – and the mother's – point of view that may have been the best outcome' (lecture to the Conservative Political Centre in Blackpool, cited in the *Sunday Telegraph*, 10 October 1993). At the same conference, John Major, the Prime Minister, coined his 'back to basics' slogan, advocating, among other things, a return to traditional teaching and respect for family values.

The confident launching of the multi-faceted attack on lone mothers and absent fathers by the Conservative government was followed by an unexpected counter-attack. At a general level, this was partly because members of the government failed to recognize that, while censure of lone mothers has historically been relatively easy to mobilize, this is no longer the case. Two specific factors account for this. First, demographic shifts in lone parenting have increased the number of people resistant to being constructed (or having their friends and relatives constructed) by the government as 'Other'. This opposition has been heightened by revelations that the private lives of some high-ranking members of that government have been inconsistent with 'back to basics'. Second, alternative, informed constructions of lone parenting are available that highlight the lack of success of policies resulting from Conservative discourses.

### Demographic changes and resistance to being constructed as Other

Over the last two decades there has been a marked increase in the percentage of all households with dependent children that consist of children with a lone mother (from 7 per cent in 1971 to 18 per cent in 1991, with lone fathers remaining at 1 per cent; Burghes 1993). This means that the appeal to 'commonplaces' was always likely to misfire. At any one time more than a million women are lone mothers, and since it is not a static state, even more women will have been or know that they are likely to become lone mothers. Many women thus pass through lone motherhood. Numerous other people know women they are related to or friendly with who are lone mothers, while many men are the fathers of the children being reared by lone mothers.

Since it is unlikely that anyone appreciates being blamed for the ills of society or being constructed as Other, the demographic shift in lone motherhood is likely to have diminished the constituency of those who support the government's 'family agenda'. In addition, such shifts are likely to reflect social changes in ideology, away from those espoused in Conservative family policies as well as changes in social practices. Those in the sub-category who are most often constructed as concrete examples of the evils of lone motherhood – teenage, never-married women (the ultimate lone mothers) – also do not consider themselves to be problematic.

When asked, 21 months after giving birth, how they thought they were coping as mothers, nearly two-thirds of the women in a London-based study of 16–19-year-old first-time mothers (reported in Phoenix 1991) said that they felt they were coping 'quite well' with their children, and just under a third said that they were coping 'very well'. More than four-fifths considered themselves to be coping as well as they wanted to with motherhood. This did not mean that they gave only glowing accounts of how they were coping. Willard Williams (1990) found that women in her US sample of black mothers under 20 were generally realistic about the demands of child care. This was also a finding in the London study of 16–19 year-old first-time mothers.

This did not mean that they rejected constructions of 'young mothers' as problematic. They did not, however, include themselves (or the people they knew and liked) in the deviant category. So, for example, mothers under 20 sometimes described other mothers in the same situation as themselves as problematic in a number of ways while, by contrast, they constructed themselves as deserving and honourable. This was sometimes a racialized construction. For example, although some council housing departments have been found to be racially discriminatory against black people (Commission for Racial Equality 1984), some white respondents said that black people were treated unfairly well when it came to getting council housing. Long waits for council housing increased some women's feelings of competitiveness with other council tenants. Similarly, women in straitened financial circumstances (many of whom lived in council housing) sometimes resented other welfare claimants.

The statements that some women made about other welfare claimants directly fitted into discourses that stigmatize 'teenage mothers' and 'lone mothers' even as they distanced themselves from the associated stigma. Thus some of the women interviewed readily reproduced existing stereotypes of lone mothers (but not themselves) becoming pregnant for instrumental reasons. In doing so, they drew on contradictory notions: that 'young mothers' are feckless, but that some young women, particularly themselves, make good, deserving mothers. This indicates that old ideologies do not necessarily disappear when people's own circumstances or experiences appear to contradict them. Instead, they sediment into common sense, making contrary themes available in everyday talk (Billig 1991). The availability of contrary themes about lone mothers, and hence their differentiation, was partially responsible for the failure of the discourse of 'lone motherhood as major social problem' to achieve the consensus expected by the Conservative government.

In any case, although over 80 per cent of women who give birth in their teenage years are single when they do so; they constitute only about 4 per cent of all lone mothers (43,500 in 1991, Babb 1993). Thus, focusing on them as the 'ultimate Others' (Brah 1993) is not likely to produce consensus that lone motherhood is generally problematic.

It is not only people constructed as deviant who exempt themselves from pathological categories while not dispensing with notions that people with similar characteristics to themselves are deviant. When Virginia Bottomley, then Secretary of State for Health, was revealed to have been a lone mother when aged 19 and a university student, the Conservative government joined ranks to refute allegations that she could be compared with irresponsible lone mothers. Timothy Yeo, then a Conservative minister, was revealed to have fathered a child outside his marriage at a time when the Conservative 'back to basics' campaign was making sexual and family values part of a moral crusade. Yeo argued that he would be contributing to his child's upbringing and hence was not an errant father (although he had helped to create a lone-mother household). Similar arguments were put forward by Cecil Parkinson when, as a minister in the Thatcher government, he was also revealed to have fathered a child by a woman other than his wife. However, both Yeo and Parkinson eventually had to resign their government positions, partly because of media outcry against the hypocrisy they demonstrated. It is perhaps not surprising that (white) middle-class fathers who are unused to being constructed as problematic are resistant to being constructed as Other by being 'pursued' by the Child Support Agency. This is particularly the case since being constructed as *refusing* to pay is rather less morally justifiable than being unable to pay.

Various Conservative Members of Parliament have blamed a range of constituencies for the increase in lone motherhood, including the church, 'politically correct' ideas and a feminist movement that 'has given encouragement to the concept that it is all right to have a child and bring the child up on your own' (Tom Sackville, Health Minister, *Guardian*, 6 July 1993). By doing so they have ostracized a range of people, some of whom might otherwise have been supportive of the 'family values' agenda.

### Alternative constructions of 'the problem' and policy failures

Discussions of lone motherhood often fit a normalized absence/pathologized presence couplet (Phoenix 1987), where those lone mothers and their children who are faring well are not discussed while those who are considered problematic make headlines. Negative discourses are bolstered by the few pieces of research that provide them with support. For example, a great deal of media attention has been given to Dennis and Erdos's (1992) report of a positive correlation between 'absent fatherhood' and levels of crime. There is, however, little evidence that lone mothers make inadequate, irresponsible parents. For example, a study by Kinsey (1993) directly contradicted the Dennis and Erdos (1992) findings. Kinsey found that children from lone-parent households, dependent on welfare, actually committed far fewer crimes than those from lone-parent households in employment.

The solutions proposed by the government to the problems they identify have been both contradictory and unsuccessful. Contradictions are demonstrated by the fact that, in May 1994, one minister, Baroness Cumberlege, advocated the provision of condoms to 12-year-olds in order to help meet the government *Health of the Nation* targets of reducing births to the under-twenties. In the same week, another minister, John Patten, advocated the tightening up of school sex education so that 'innocent'/ignorant children are protected from knowledge and not given sexually explicit information. Similarly, policies designed to reduce the entitlement to council housing of lone mothers run counter to ideologies of child protection and children's rights to be adequately provided for. The controversies generated by the operation of the Child Support Agency (which did have cross-party support) is a case of government lack of preparedness for problems that had been brought to their attention by pressure groups. The potential benefits of the Act for lone mothers have, according to Sue Slipman (1993), then director of the National Council for One Parent Families (NCOPF), not been realized because of inept implementation.

While government policies on lone mothers have been demonstrably unsuccessful, there has been, in recent years, an increase in research, the findings of which take issue with dominant notions that lone motherhood is, in itself, a problem. Work by Millar (1989, 1995), Bradshaw and Millar (1991), Hardey and Crow (1991) and Burghes (1993) indicate that, far from living in luxury on welfare payments, lone mothers are struggling in poverty. The policy options that these researchers suggest are based on research findings and aim to reduce the dependence of lone mothers on state benefits (something that many lone mothers themselves would welcome) while increasing their incomes.

## THE ABSENCE OF 'RACE': THE CASE OF THE SILENT DISCOURSE

Black families have consistently been identified as problematic in both Britain and the USA (McAdoo 1988; Phoenix 1987, 1990, 1993). In particular, high rates of lone motherhood in populations of African origin have been blamed for problems ranging from educational underachievement to delinquency (see, for example, the report of the official inquiry into the underachievement of 'West Indian' children in British schools, which focuses on the high rates of lone parenthood among 'West Indian' families; Swann 1985). High rates of lone motherhood have been an important focus in the construction of black families as outside the British nation (Gilroy 1987). In addition, US theories of the underclass have focused on self-perpetuating groups of alienated, unemployed men who engage in criminal activities but do not participate in family life with the young women with whom they produce children (Wilson 1987). These theories have generated concern about the high percentage of 'the underclass' that is black. In the United States, concerns about lone mothers continue to be racialized (Morris 1994). Given the historical pervasiveness of pathological constructions of black lone mothers (Lawrence 1982), it might be expected that recent discourses of lone motherhood in Britain would be particularly aimed at black mothers of African-

Caribbean origin. This is not, however, the case. In the current moral panic about lone parenting there has been, apparently, no explicit attempt to link 'race' and nation with lone motherhood.

The absence of discourses of black pathology in recent constructions of lone motherhood is so strikingly obvious that it requires explanation. Scott-Jones and Nelson-Le Gall (1986) argue that social issues perceived to pertain to minority ethnic groups are generally not taken seriously. If, however, white majorities start behaving in the same way, the issue comes to be seen as less problematic, but also generally gets taken more seriously. Arguably then, while lone motherhood was seen as almost exclusively a black aberration, it was censured, but constructed as due to cultural difference and the Otherness of black people (Phoenix 1990, 1991). Over the last two decades a handful of writers have argued that similar behaviours in black and white 'young', single mothers necessarily have different aetiologies. Thus, in a review of US literature, Phipps-Yonas (1980) pointed out that individualistic, psychological explanations tended to be advanced in explanation of pregnancies to single, white young women, whereas 'cultural reasons' tended to be advanced in explanation of black 'teenage pregnancies'. The few pieces of British work attempting to explain black and white differences in rates of lone 'teenage motherhood' have racialized the issues in similar ways, constructing white and black lone 'teenage motherhood' as the result respectively of individual aberration and group cultural norms (Phoenix 1988).

Rickie Solinger (1994) argues that, while there have been historical shifts in the ways in which 'illegitimacy' is constructed in the United States, black and white 'illegitimate' babies have, particularly since the 1940s, been constructed differently. 'In short, after World War II, the white bastard child was no longer the child nobody wanted. The Black illegitimate baby became the child white politicians and taxpayers loved to hate' (Solinger 1994: 287). Thus, black lone mothers were expected to keep their babies, while white lone mothers were expected to give up their babies for adoption. In this construction, black lone mothers were constructed as irredeemably Other, while white lone mothers could experience redemption by relinquishing their babies.

The benign neglecters began to articulate their position at about the same time that the psychologists provided new explanations for white single pregnancy. In tandem, these developments set Black and white unwed mothers in different universes of cause and effect . . . . Thus, by becoming mothers, even unwed mothers, Black women were simply doing what came naturally. There was no reason for social service workers or policymakers to interfere. Since professionals could have an impact on the immediate situation – and could not penetrate or rearrange Black 'culture,' it was doubly futile to consider interfering.

(Solinger 1994: 298–9)

While high rates of lone motherhood seemed confined to black populations in the United States and Britain, 'cultural' explanations of black lone motherhood were largely unquestioned. However, as white women have increasingly become lone mothers over the last decade, the assumption of necessary black and white differences in family forms has increasingly been shown to be inadequate. Furstenberg, Brooks-Gunn and Morgan (1987) are among those who have had to re-evaluate black and white differences and commonalities in patterns of lone motherhood as white young women have started to show patterns similar to those associated with black young women:

By the mid-1980s, almost all children of black teenage mothers were born out-of-wedlock. . . . These dramatic changes helped create the belief that teenage childbearing is primarily a black issue. But recent trends suggest that blacks may simply have been pacesetters for the population at large.

(Furstenberg et al. 1987: 5)

There is, currently, a great deal of work (from a variety of perspectives) that attempts to explain lone motherhood in black populations (see, for example, Dickerson 1995). How then can the absence of mention of black lone mothers in recent British Conservative discourses on lone motherhood be explained?

Demography may be argued to provide one explanation for the lack of racialization of discourses of lone motherhood. For black lone mothers currently constitute a tiny percentage of all lone mothers. In fact, on the basis of figures from the 1991 British census, about half of black mothers of African-Caribbean origin in Britain are lone parents at any one time (C. Owen, personal communication 1995). However, people of African-Caribbean descent constitute less than 1 per cent of the British population. There is also more employment among black women than among white women (D. Owen 1994), making black lone mothers less likely than white lone mothers to be dependent on state provision. As a result, there is little point in aiming censure particularly at black lone mothers if government aim is to reduce welfare payments. The appeal has to be wider, going beyond black mothers. However, governments are not noted for paying particular attention to demographic trends or always using statistics accurately and responsibly when formulating policy decisions or making rallying speeches. This is evident in the debate about the figures cited by John Redwood to warrant his concern about high rates of single parent-hood on the St Mellon's estate in Wales in 1993. These figures were reproduced in a BBC *Panorama* programme on lone mothers. A complaint was subsequently made by the National Council for One Parent Families (NCOPF) which included a refutation of the figures used by Redwood and *Panorama*. The NCOPF cited research commissioned by South Glamorgan Social Services, and conducted by Pithouse *et al.* (1991) at the University of Cardiff, to argue that less than 20 per cent of parents in the area Redwood was talking about (St Mellon's) were actually lone parents (compared to the 65 per cent that Redwood claimed). Despite the accusations of having used inaccurate figures, neither Redwood nor the *Panorama* programme retracted their statements. In addition, as Seidman and Rappoport (1986) argue, it is common for the construction of social problems to be characterized by 'generalizations from extreme samples'. In keeping with this, black lone mothers have frequently been stereotyped as 'typical' lone mothers (Ziegler 1995).

A further explanation could be argued to be the disruption of the assumed link between family structure and the lawless behaviour of black male youth of African-Caribbean descent. The disruption of this link is important to a consideration of lone motherhood, since it has been commonplace for social scientists as well as politicians to blame the perceived ills of black young people (poor educational attainment as well as lawlessness) on 'female-headed households' and 'father absence'.

> The point implied in much of the literature is that a lot of the culturally 'abnormal' behaviour of minority groups can be traced back to supposed family deficiencies. Additionally, the proble-matic black family background is often implicated in explanations for unrest, decay, and violence in the inner cities.
>
> (Brittan and Maynard 1984: 34)

Scarman's discussion of the black community in the Brixton area [following his official inquiry into the Brixton 'riots'] . . . begins with a section on the family which reproduces the stereotyped image of black household beset by generational conflict and torn asunder by antagonism between authoritarian parents.... The pathological character of these households is established in the text by a discussion of the effects of male absence and of male presence.... According to Scarman, the resulting 'matriarchy' undergoes 'destructive changes' under the impact of British social conditions and the disintegration of this basic structure of life is part of the chain reaction which ended in the Brixton riot.

(Gilroy 1987: 104–5)

In the 1990s, various clashes between the British police and public have made it less tenable to assert that modern urban disorder is only the province of young black masculinity. The clashes have occurred on predominantly white council housing estates in Newcastle, on mixed estates in Luton, with Asian youth in Bradford, with white young people attending rave parties and with travellers. Despite this, however, the assumed link between 'race' and crime has not disappeared. A letter from the Commissioner of the Metropolitan Police, Sir Paul Condon, to black 'community leaders', leaked to the British press in July 1995, argued that most muggings are committed by 'very young black people... excluded from school'. However, it made no mention of black families, lone or otherwise, as causally responsible. Nor has the debate generated by this leak focused on the black families from which these 'muggers' come. Is it then the case that Conservatives have not censured black lone mothers because it is no longer plausible to suggest that black families are mainly responsible for urban unrest? Has the space created by the silencing of discourses on the deviance of black lone-parent families been filled by discourses on the deviance of some white families, in particular those headed by lone mothers?

Such a conclusion is unwarranted. Michael Keith in discussing a London newspaper's 1990 description of 'typical muggers' argues that their description is racialized although there is no explicit statement about 'race'. 'The identikit rioter, the alienated criminal, the designer mugger; there is no need to say *they* are Black because *we* already know it' (Keith 1993: 248). In a similar way, the fact that there are long-standing and pervasive linkages between black lone-parent families and black male crime in discourses of 'law and order' makes it unnecessary for black young men's assumed criminality to be blamed explicitly on black family structure. The link has already been made and so is already known. The historical location of 'the problem' of lone parenthood is such that 'we already know' that the worst offenders with regard to lone motherhood are black lone mothers. The already established 'commonplace' no longer needs to be spelled out (Billig 1991). While Conservative discourses would probably not be taken seriously by white lone parents if they were aimed specifically at black lone parents, it is extremely easy for old racialized constructions to become evident and, hence, to be demonstrated to be still in operation. Ziegler (1995) illustrates this with a high-profile example from the United States where, in 1992, Dan Quayle, then the Republican vice-president, attacked 'Murphy Brown', a character in a television soap opera, for choosing to become a lone mother:

> It is ironic that Quayle chose to pick on TV character Murphy Brown, who is portrayed as a single woman with an annual income of more than $50,000 who made the choice to be a single parent, because Murphy does not fit the typical stereotype usually associated with single parenting, primarily and often profiled as an African American female who is on welfare. As a matter of fact, on the evening of the sitcom's 1992 fall premiers where Murphy struck back at the vice-president, Quayle selected a group of African American single parents in Washington DC, to view the program with him to serve as a symbol of his support for single parenting. Unfortunately, Quayle's choice of this racial composition for the audience opened the door for more comments regarding his motives.
>
> (Ziegler 1995: 81)

Quayle's choice of black lone mothers to view the programme with him was widely interpreted as a blunder. For while he had never explicitly criticized black single parents, his gesture was interpreted by many to give a coded racial message about who he considered as 'typical' lone parents.

The implicit racialization of discourses of lone motherhood intersects with the racialization of insider–outsider status with regard to the British nation in a way that contributes to explanations of the absence of 'race' in recent discourses of lone motherhood. Black families have long been constructed as outsiders in the British nation. A central tenet of 'new racism' in political discourses has been the counterposing of threatening hordes of often lawless black people, who, if allowed, would 'swamp' British society, with the construction of Britain as consisting of a homogeneous culture (Barker 1981). The discourses and policies aimed at black people that result from these constructions are related to immigration controls and rights of citizenship. A statement from Margaret Thatcher, in the period just before her first election as British Prime Minister, which was delivered in a television interview, clearly constructs black populations as a threat from without. 'People really are rather afraid that this country might be swamped by people with a different culture' (Margaret Thatcher, *Daily Mail*, January 1978).

There have been recurrent demands by British politicians and the media that 'foreigners' and outsiders should be excluded from claims to British social security payments. Some lone mothers, who cannot be positioned as outside the nation, have also been subjected to proclamations that they should be prevented from making 'dishonest' welfare claims. Peter Lilley, the Conservative Social Security Secretary, has repeatedly advocated a 'crackdown' on 'fraudulent' welfare claims made, according to him, by one in five lone parents living on welfare (Brindle 1995b). Highlighting the lawlessness of large numbers of lone parents is a strategy for generating consensus about the problematic nature of lone mothers. However, such pronouncements cannot be applied to those lone parents who are 'insiders' in the British nation, and who claim only those benefits the state has decreed that they are entitled to receive. In that context, it makes little sense to include those constructed as necessarily outside the supposedly unitary British culture in discourses of lone motherhood. Outsiders' claims are constructed as unauthorized in other ways. Instead, lone parents, particularly those who attempt to defraud the British state, have been constructed as the threat from *within* the British nation:

> Children are in danger of seeing life without the father, not as the exception, but as the rule. This is a new kind of threat to our way of life, the long term implications of which we cannot grasp.
>
> (Margaret Thatcher, Speech to the National Children's Home, 1990)

The discourses of black and of white lone motherhood thus do not converge and cannot easily be reconciled. On the one hand, discourses about black lone mothers construct those who have been held to be responsible for many of the ills considered to beset black people and white society as Other and outsiders from British society. Their high rates of lone motherhood are thus constructed as the threat from outside the nation. On the other hand, white lone mothers are insiders in the British nation, but are constructed as constituting a threat from within, outsiders with regard to 'normal' and responsible parenting behaviour. Solinger (1994) found a historical differentiation in the United States between constructions of black and white 'illegitimacy':

> Black, unmarried mothers, in contrast, were said to offer bad value (Black babies) at a high price (taxpayer-supported welfare grants) to the detriment of society, demographically and economically....The fact that it was, overwhelmingly, a buyers' market for Black babies 'proved' the valuelessness of these children, despite their expense to the taxpaying public. White babies entered a healthy sellers' market, with up to ten couples competing for every one adoptable infant.
>
> (Solinger 1994: 300)

The incompatibility of the discourses of insiders and of outsiders provides a central reason that black lone mothers have not been targeted in speeches designed to reduce support for welfare provision for lone mothers. It is insiders, whose belonging to the nation cannot easily be challenged, who are the targets in such campaigns. The omission of lone black mothers in this instance still renders them pathological since it indicates that they are not genuinely British. Leaving 'race' silent in recent discourses of lone motherhood thus does not signify the deracialization of such discourses. As such it leaves open the possibility that 'race' can be directly invoked, when necessary, in future discourses of lone motherhood.

## CONCLUSION

The ways in which the British Conservative government of the mid-1990s focused on lone motherhood as a social problem has not produced fruitful solutions. This is partly due to the failure to distinguish between different groups of lone mothers while making the most dramatic case by treating all lone mothers as if they are young and single: generalizing from extreme samples. Inappropriate solutions have resulted from the narrow constructions favoured by Conservative politicians and have, in addition, reduced popular support for government pronouncements. Assumptions that it is easy to appeal to 'commonplaces' about 'the family' have proved unfounded, as lone motherhood has proved to be a contested terrain characterized by contradictory social constructions.

Over the last three decades there have been both demographic and ideological shifts related to lone motherhood. It has proved difficult for a government that has asserted itself strongly with regard to policies on 'the family' to accommodate to changes in discursive constructions, particularly since 'the family' is a favoured site for policy implementation. This makes contradictions and conflicts in government discourses and policies apparent. Inadequate definitions of what is problematic about lone motherhood have led to simplistic and ineffective solutions that often perpetuate the problems they were designed to solve, rather than alleviating the poverty faced by the majority of lone mothers and addressed in various studies.

The absence of specific discourses on black lone mothers in recent Conservative government discourses appears welcome, but results from the targeting of those constructed as problematic *within* the nation. Since black families are constructed as *outsiders* in the nation, their current absence from discourses against lone motherhood is indicative of the exclusion of black families from Conservative constructions of the British nation.

# Chapter 11

# Unpalatable choices and inadequate families

Lone mothers and the underclass debate

*Sasha Roseneil and Kirk Mann*

Alongside the growth in the number of women both having children outside marriage and bringing them up alone, recent years have seen extensive public debate about lone motherhood. This chapter explores the way this debate has created a category of mothers that is not only deemed 'not good enough' at the raising of children but is also pinpointed as positively harmful to society. Our particular focus is on the powerful and widespread discourse that gripped the media and policy circles in the early 1990s; this discourse links lone motherhood with the creation and reproduction of an 'underclass' in contemporary society. While this period is certainly not unique in its concern about the breakdown of 'the family' and the rise in the number of never-married mothers, this specific discursive construction of lone motherhood is particularly interesting. The intensity of media interest and the prolific nature of government pronouncements and policy proposals on the subject suggest that the confluence of the issue of lone motherhood with the notion that there is a dangerous and growing underclass has taken a firm hold on the collective conscience of British and US society.

In this chapter we explore why this discourse about lone mothers, absent fathers and the underclass has achieved such widespread credibility. Our focus is primarily on its expression in Britain, though we identify its origins in the United States, and we pass comment on the differing courses it has taken on each side of the Atlantic. We attempt to unravel some of the complex threads of moral concerns about the decline of the family, fiscal concerns about welfare benefits and 'the costs' of dependency, and a largely unspoken, but lurking, anti-feminism. We suggest that this discourse is located within the framework of a welfare state that is in the process of restructuring, and within a wider project of 'patriarchal reconstruction' (Smart 1989), and that it constitutes a 'backlash' against long-term changes in gender relations and against feminism. Towards the end of the chapter we take up an issue that is at the heart of the discourse but has largely been ignored by other feminist and critical commentators: the question of agency.

## 1993: THE YEAR OF THE LONE MOTHER

Our initial interest was prompted by the widespread moral outrage that followed the murder of a 2-year-old boy, James Bulger, in February 1993. In the period that followed the murder, the media homed in on lone mothers and their fatherless, supposedly criminally inclined children, identifying them as the core of the underclass and the source of many contemporary social problems. Although the intensity of this 'moral panic' ebbed in the months that followed, 1993 was, in many respects, 'the year of the lone mother' in Britain. The press, tabloid and broadsheet alike, was full of articles about the 'problem' of never-married mothers, and television and radio documentaries and discussion programmes were devoted to the topic. For the second year running, the Conservative Party conference in the Autumn of 1993 rang to denunciations of single mothers, and an ill-fated 'back to basics' programme to restore the nation's morality was launched.[1]

The discourse about the underclass that developed in 1993 dichotomized women along age-old lines – good women who do the right thing, get married and then have children, versus bad women, who have children, don't get married and depend on state benefits. By the second half of the year, attention was not just on the social costs of fatherless families that fail properly to socialize their children but included the financial costs as well.

As Smart (Chapter 2 of this volume, and 1992) and many other writers have documented, the problematization of unmarried mothers (who are consistently condemned more than mothers who are single through divorce, abandonment or widowhood) has a long history and has, at different times, emphasized variously the economic, the moral and the psychological problems caused by lone mothers.[2] Moral outrage about lone mothers, particularly young mothers, existed throughout the 1980s (McRobbie 1989; Phoenix 1991), and it had been escalating from 1987 (Fox Harding 1993a). In 1991 the media erupted in a brief furore about 'virgin births', as evidence that growing numbers of women, particularly lesbians, were becoming 'lone mothers by choice', and doing so without even sexual contact with men (Radford 1991). Despite this history, there are good reasons for seeing developments in 1993 as novel.

First, the level of political vitriol against lone mothers, particularly never-married mothers, reached a new intensity by 1993; the speeches of Ministers Lilley and Redwood seized the headlines on numerous occasions and whipped the Tory faithful into ecstatic applause. Second, the context within which the discourse was produced was different from that pertaining during previous outbreaks of outrage about lone mothers. Throughout the 1980s there was a significant increase in the proportion of families headed by never-married mothers; by the beginning of the 1990s, 27 per cent of births were to unmarried mothers, with especially high rates in some areas (for example, 54 per cent in North Manchester; Muncie *et al.* 1995). Of course, many of these mothers will get married, may be in a heterosexual relationship already, or will not be intending to rely on single-parent benefits. Nevertheless, we would suggest that a significant minority of lone mothers do not intend to marry and see no place in their families for a 'father figure' (see, for example, Renvoize 1985; Morris 1992; Gordon 1990, 1994). While this may have been true of a very small proportion of lone mothers in the past, there appears to be a new confidence and assertiveness in many women. For many, despite the difficulties associated with lone motherhood, there seems to be a pragmatic feeling that they can manage, albeit with state support, and that the father is an obstacle to a stable life for themselves and their children. These women are not necessarily 'abandoned' by the fathers, nor should their pregnancies be assumed to be 'accidents'; in this respect, they are not victims.

The final reason why the 1993 discourse about lone mothers is significant is that it was disseminated extremely widely throughout the media. It dominated the political agenda to an unprecedented extent and elicited a considerable degree of consensus across the left–right political divide. With its differing strands, emphasizing morality or economics, the discourse united Tory traditionalists concerned with 'family values' and morality, Christian socialists and liberals with similar interests, and Thatcherite hardliners keen to continue 'rolling back the welfare state'. Moreover, and in contrast to earlier panics about the morality of young women, events in 1993 enabled these groups to engage with each other. Above all, the authority of the discourse rested on the status of two of its leading exponents – the American, Charles Murray (1990), and the Briton, A.H. Halsey (1992).

## MORAL PANIC: JUVENILE CRIME AND THE PROBLEM CHILDREN OF PROBLEM MOTHERS

As Hall *et al.* (1978) point out, a widespread 'moral panic' about the 'steadily rising rate of violent crime' has been simmering away in British society since the 1960s. The most recent outbreak of moral indignation began with a focus on car crime committed by young men, and the racing of stolen cars around council estates drew widespread media coverage in 1991.

However, media attention to juvenile crime reached unprecedented heights in February 1993 following the murder of James Bulger. Still photographs from security video cameras in the mall showed the child with two figures, who appeared to be in their early teens. A hunt began for the murderers, during which several teenage boys were arrested and then eventually released uncharged. When two 10-year-old boys finally appeared in court, a crowd of about 250 people gathered outside, many hurling missiles and abuse at the accused (*Guardian*, 23 February 1993).

The concern about juvenile crime that crystalized around the Bulger case can be labelled a 'moral panic', given the unanimity with which police, politicians, journalists and sections of the public reacted 'out of all proportion to the actual threat' (Hall *et al.* 1978: 16). Initially the panic concerned juvenile crime, but later it transpired that the 'real', underlying problem was lone mothers. From the breaking of the news about the murder of James Bulger until several weeks after the charging of suspects, the issue of juvenile crime dominated the media. The commentary of 'experts' and the 'vox pop' of the general public saturated the press, television and radio, all discussing the 'new' phenomenon of serious juvenile crime. From one murder, within the background context of rising car crime, was extrapolated a major new social scourge.

Condemnation of juvenile crime was not limited to those traditionally vocal on issues of law and order; indeed, the Labour Party made much of the running in the aftermath of the Bulger murder, with Tony Blair, soon-to-be Labour Party Leader, declaring Labour policy to be 'tough on crime, and tough on the causes of crime' (*Guardian*, 22 February 1993).

The gender politics of this moral panic about juvenile crime emerge in the analyses proffered by the media and by those 'experts' asked to explain the phenomenon. Despite Prime Minister John Major's declaration that society should 'condemn a little more and understand a little less', a veritable industry of pop sociology emerged during the lifetime of the panic. Both Murray and Halsey, appearing in the *Sunday Times* and the *Guardian* respectively, along with editorials in almost every newspaper, linked the phenomenon of juvenile crime with the emergence of an underclass in British society, and this with the breakdown of the nuclear family and the increase in births outside marriage. Rising juvenile crime was presented as both the evidence and the result of a growing underclass composed primarily of never-married mothers and their children. The solution to the problem therefore (sometimes implicit, other times explicit) was simple: the reconstitution of the nuclear family and the reassertion of the power and role of the father within it (e.g. Halsey 1992, Murray 1990).

## UNPALATABLE CHOICES AND INADEQUATE FAMILIES

Although Murray does not reflect the views of any sizeable academic constituency in Britain, he is an important and influential figure. In 1987 he had meetings with Department of Health and Social Security and Treasury officials and members of the then Prime Minister's Policy Unit, and two years later he addressed the Prime Minister (Dean and Taylor-Gooby 1992: 5). The press are not generally noted for their keen interest in the work of social scientists, but the views of Murray have been invoked to provide academic credibility for various leader writers and social commentators. The *Sunday Times* has persistently cited Murray, with Andrew Neil, the paper's former editor, pointing out that it was his newspaper that introduced Murray to the British public and sponsored his 'research' in Britain in 1989. Murray's ideas have also been disseminated by News International Group newspapers in other countries. Right-wing think tanks – the Institute of Economic Affairs in Britain and the Centre for Industrial Studies in Australia – have been quick to adopt Murray's arguments, both publishing his work (Murray 1990), and imprinting their other publications with the mark of his theories (e.g. Dennis and Erdos 1992; Davies 1993). Thus, and despite the fact that he has done little primary research, Murray has found a receptive international audience and a number of followers among journalists and politicians. As an American, Murray is considered to be well placed to tell Britain what the future may hold if unmarried mothers are allowed to continue reproducing the underclass unchecked. Comparisons with the United States are commonplace within the British discourse, with the spectre of American inner-city social dislocation and violence given prominence (MacGregor 1990).[3]

According to Murray, there are three types of behaviour associated with membership of the underclass: illegitimacy, violent crime and drop-out from the labour force. He does not make clear whether these forms of behaviour are cause or consequence of underclass membership. What is clear, however, is that the underclass, to put it in the 'common-sense' language Murray is so fond of, is composed of 'idle, thieving bastards' (Bagguley and Mann 1992).

Like many right-wing observers, Murray presents the issue in terms of rational choices. Whereas choice is usually portrayed by the right as a tremendous benefit to society and the economy, it is seen as inappropriate for women who want to have children without the support of an economically active man. Thus David Green of the Institute of Economic Affairs (in the Institute's series entitled 'Choice in Welfare') laments the fact that, 'The traditional family of mum, dad and the kids has become just another lifestyle choice.' He goes on to ask, 'Is every moral value just another lifestyle option? Or is there a minimum stock of values which we ignore at our peril?' (Green 1993: vi).

Never-married mothers are deemed to have made the wrong choices, albeit, according to Murray, rational ones. Murray argues that lone mothers choose dependence on the state in preference to marriage because the benefit system privileges the lone mother over the two-parent family. This combines with the fact that there is no longer a stigma to illegitimacy to mean that many young women no longer see the need to marry in order to have children. Murray goes on to suggest that these women are denying their children suitable masculine role models and denying young men a respectable role as father figures. There is a moral vacuum, it is claimed, which has its roots in the 'permissive society' of the 1960s, the period when Murray detects a shift in social values. The stigma that Murray feels is so important in deterring illegitimacy was eroded by the 'sexual revolution of the 1960s' (Murray 1990: 28). As he says:

> There is an obvious explanation for why single young women get pregnant: sex is fun and babies endearing. Nothing could be more

natural than for young men and women to have sex, and nothing could be more natural than for a young woman to want to have a baby.

(Murray 1990: 28)

Only the financial restraints of subsistence benefits and social opprobrium can restrain such biologically determined, natural inclinations. In Murray's world view both men and women are driven by essential impulses – men to reckless barbarian behaviour and promiscuous sex, women to reproduction and motherhood. In order for society to function smoothly, this Hobbesian state of nature must be tamed by moral codes and economic sanctions. However, he does not suggest that all 'fatherless families' are part of the underclass: widows and divorcees are generally exempt, as are affluent women with careers who choose to be unmarried lone parents. The focus is squarely on working-class women.

According to Murray, 'illegitimacy' is bad for both men and boys, and as a consequence is bad for society as a whole, whether or not it is good or bad for women does not enter his discussion. First of all, boys brought up without a male role model in female-headed households do not receive adequate socialization into manhood:

Little boys don't naturally grow up to be responsible fathers and husbands. They don't naturally grow up knowing how to get up every morning at the same time and go to work. They don't naturally grow up thinking that work is not just a way to make money, but a way to hold one's head high in the world.

(Murray 1990: 10–11)

Without a father, adolescent boys are unruly and criminal; 'in communities without fathers the kids tend to run wild. The fewer the fathers, the greater the tendency' (Murray 1990: 12).

Not being a real father, a father who works to provide for his wife and family, is also bad for adult men themselves. Paid work must be 'the centre of life' for young men.

Supporting a family is a central means for a man to prove to himself that he is a 'mensch'. Men who do not support families find other ways to prove that they are men .... [Y]oung males are essentially barbarians for whom marriage – meaning not just the wedding vows but the act of taking responsibility for a wife and children – is an indispensable civilizing force.

(Murray 1990: 23)

These views about the vital importance of fathers to social stability have since been echoed by Halsey, speaking from an 'ethical socialist' perspective:

> The very, very important ingredient of a role model of a working man, a person who goes to work and comes back and does all sorts of DIY and is a responsible adult person, is missing. And that seems to be a way of making sure you don't have barbarism. Because young men, grown men have got nothing to do with anything that really matters and they just faff around satisfying their own desires, tastes.
>
> (*Panorama*, BBC1, 20 September 1993)

Following the Bulger murder, the *Sunday Times* solicited Murray's views from the United States about the problem of juvenile crime and resurrected his earlier commentary. The marks of his theories are clearly visible in an editorial entitled 'Return of the Family':

> It is becoming increasingly clear to all but the most blinkered of social scientists that the disintegration of the nuclear family is the principal source of so much social unrest and misery. The creation of an urban underclass, on the margins of society, but doing great damage to itself and the rest of us, is directly linked to the rapid rise in illegitimacy.
>
> The past two decades have witnessed the growth of whole communities in which the dominant family structure is the single-parent mother on welfare, whose male offspring are already immersed in a criminal culture by the time they are teenagers and whose daughters are destined to follow the family tradition of unmarried mothers .... [F]or communities to function success-fully they need families with fathers.
>
> (*Sunday Times*, 28 February 1993)

Startlingly similar opinions have also been expressed in the British liberal press. Melanie Phillips in the *Guardian* had already been writing about the problem of the underclass before the juvenile crime panic erupted; the Bulger murder provided the moment for a full-scale campaign to 'rediscover the values of the family' (*Guardian*, 26 February 1993). Phillips hangs her polemic on the work of Halsey, whom she interviewed for the *Guardian* (23 February 1993). Halsey 'feels passionately that the decline of the nuclear family is not merely at the root of many social ills but is the cancer in the lungs of the modern left'. He laments the disappearance of the specificity of the 'family contract', and the absence of male role models in contemporary families:

> We're talking about a situation where the man never arrives, never mind leaves. There is a growing proportion of children born into single parent families where the father has never participated as a father but only as a genital.
>
> (*Guardian*, 23 February 1993)

Apparently Halsey feels that, without a father, the child (implicitly male), grows up unable to see women 'as anything other than objects of sexual manipulation and gratification'. (Presumably when mothers also perform domestic labour for their husbands, fathers disavow boys of the idea that women only provide sexual servicing!)

Using Halsey's ideas as academic legitimation for her own, and citing the work of the Institute for Public Policy Research, Phillips argues that being brought up by a lone mother is bad for children's psychological development. Public policy should explicitly support two-parent families, and enforce paternal responsibility.

So, the views of the conservative, Murray, and the socialist, Halsey, are remarkably close, the most obvious difference being that Halsey places considerable emphasis on the need for real men to be keen at DIY. Both commentators paint peculiarly romantic pictures of patriarchal masculinity that seem to be locked into the 1950s. But with the decline of the sort of 'respectable working-class' employment in manufacturing industry that Murray's 'mensch' would have taken, the rise in the service sector, women's employment and part-time working, their ideal family structure confronts head-on the reality of the free market in the 1990s.

## FISCAL CRISIS AND THE WELFARE STATE

By mid-1993, the lone mother was being assessed in terms of her economic as well as her moral and social costs to the nation. The *Sunday Times* (11 July 1993) again led the way for the media with a special pull-out with the following headlines across four pages: 'Wedded to Welfare'; 'Do they want to marry a man or the state?'; 'Once illegitimacy was punished – now it is rewarded'. Murray was once again provided with space to argue that there is 'no point fiddling with welfare at the margin', and that 'only marriage and the principle of legitimacy will preserve a liberal society.' The cartoon that accompanied this special pull-out – a faceless male social security officer with a pregnant bride on his arm and three children emerging from beneath her dress, a beer swilling man/father just in the background – hardly corresponded with any liberal values of tolerance. Likewise, leader comments in the *Daily Telegraph*, the *Daily Mail* and the *Daily Express* (15 July 1993) echoed Welsh Secretary John Redwood's condemnation (2 July 1993) of women who had children 'with no apparent intention of even trying marriage or a stable relationship with the father of the child' (quoted in Blackie 1994: 18).

The simple equation that was propagated was as follows: public spending is out of control, a major reason for the increase in public spending is the number of mothers on benefit, they reproduce the values of welfare dependency in their children, an underclass of such people is forming, therefore a downward spiral of moral decline and an upward spiral of welfare costs is the future that Britain faces.

Lone mothers were not the only group relying on public welfare to be the target of critical comments, but they were seen as one of the 'softer' political targets.[4] As the debate within the Conservative Party over how to tackle the public debt intensified, attention that had already that year been focused on lone mothers as the producers of the underclass was harnessed in their direction once more. Speeches in July 1993 about the economic burden of never-married mothers occurred shortly after a seminar organized by the Institute of Economic Affairs, which attracted some of those who were subsequently so vocal on the topic.

Apart from the work of Murray, whose research consisted of little more than a trawl through some existing secondary sources and a few conversations with interesting 'characters', the media were not interested in existing research. While Murray was held up as a beacon of academic integrity and Halsey as someone who had seen the light, and Phillips lambasted social scientists for failing to research the problems, there was no interest in work that contradicted Murray. No one quoted Macnicol (1987), who has pointed out that in the past it was common for observers to discuss 'the dangerous classes', the 'residuum' and their 'culture of poverty', but that these notions have been discredited in recent years. Likewise, and despite the fact that the United States was so often the 'nightmare' haunting Britain, no one thought it worth quoting William Prosser, Senior Policy Advisor to President Bush, who dismissed the underclass idea as little more than a reworking of older, discredited, concepts like the culture of poverty (Prosser 1990; Mann 1992). More recent empirical work, such as that of Dean and Taylor-Gooby, which shows that lone parents hold views that 'adhere to the mainstream values of work and family ethics' (Dean and Taylor-Gooby 1992: 5), were never mentioned. Rather, the press used 'common sense' to ride roughshod over complex social issues and changes. The facts that the average duration of lone parenthood for never-married mothers is only 35 months (Ermisch 1986), that many lone mothers may live in fear of the child's father, and that the majority of lone mothers are not 'single' but divorced or separated (Brown 1989) were rarely reflected in the press.

## ANTI-LONE MOTHER DISCOURSE IN BRITAIN AND THE UNITED STATES

Although much of the preceding discussion is unique to Britain in the early 1990s, there are many parallels with the United States. In both countries there has been a concerted ideological offensive against the welfare state by radical conservatives, and in both countries lone mothers have been highlighted as a serious financial burden on the taxpayer. Murray's analysis, which he developed in the 1980s, was exported from the United States pretty much wholesale to Britain, and with this came suggestions that Britain adopt policies such as the New Jersey scheme that refuses benefit to women who have a second child while still dependent on welfare.

However, there are two substantial differences between anti-lone-mother rhetoric in Britain and in the United States. First, in the USA the discourse has long been racialized in a manner almost completely absent in Britain. Solinger argues that there are 'two histories of single pregnancy in the post-World War II era, one for Black women and one for white' (Solinger 1994: 287). Whereas white women who gave birth outside marriage increasingly became subject to a psychological discourse, which constructed them as maladjusted and in need of help, black women who did the same were seen as merely expressing their 'natural', 'unrestrained sexuality' (Solinger 1994: 299). Illegitimate white babies could therefore be removed from their mothers and adopted by 'stable' couples (thereby fulfilling the demand for white babies for adoption) on the grounds that this would both provide their mothers with the best chance of overcoming their neuroses, and at the same time offer the best future to the child. Illegitimate black babies, on the other hand, were left with their mothers, because adoption demand was less than for white babies, and because it was thought that their mothers were not in need of a 'cure'. Public discourse about lone motherhood in this period focused on black women. Southern Dixiecrats and Northern racists united to condemn the social liability of black illegitimate children, and opinion polls suggested that the American people wanted to withdraw Aid to Dependent Children from these children (Solinger 1994: 301). Black women thus became, often unwillingly, the first group in the United States to receive publicly subsidized birth control, sterilization and abortion (Ward 1986).

In the 1980s and 1990s the American discourse continued to highlight the special 'problem' of black lone motherhood. With the conservatives to the fore, liberal commentators increasingly acquiesced in the growing consensus that 'something did have to be done about the offspring of the (mainly black) underclass, who, raised by teen moms, grow into gun-wielding, benefit-draining, drug-dealing hoodlums' (*Guardian*, 31 January 1995). To date, black women have not been specifically targeted in Britain in the same way as in the United States (see Chapter 10 by Phoenix in this volume).

The second difference between the discourse in the United States and Britain is that it has achieved far greater hegemony in the USA. Both countries have seen the highest increases in lone motherhood in the developed world (Chandler 1991), but rates, particularly for lone mothers under 20, remain higher in the USA (Phoenix 1991). This, combined with the far greater political and cultural strength of the right in the USA, has meant that the discourse has been pushed further there than in Britain. In 1994, the Republicans regained control of Congress on the basis of their 'Contract with America', which promised to eradicate 'the culture of welfare dependency'. Two major planks in the programme of the Republican speaker of the House, Newt Gingrich, both constitute attacks on lone motherhood: the 'American Dream Restoration Act', which will provide tax credits for two-parent families, and the proposal to remove children from their unmarried mothers and place them in orphanages, in order to break the cycle by which the underclass is reproduced (*Guardian*, 26 November 1994, 31 January 1995). In Britain, in contrast, although 'discrimination' against couples with children and in favour of lone parents in the allocation of council (state-subsidized) housing has been condemned by government ministers, the policy response has been to remove the obligation on local authorities to give priority to all the statutorily homeless in the allocation of housing. This move will disproportionately affect lone mothers, but is not aimed exclusively at them, suggesting that it has been more difficult to translate political rhetoric into policy proposals in Britain than it has been, and probably will be, in the United States.

## ANTI-FEMINIST BACKLASH

Thus far our analysis of why the 1990s has seen such widespread concern about lone mothers has focused on the moral panic that erupted over the issue of juvenile crime and the targeting of lone mothers as part of the ideologically and fiscally motivated restructuring of the British welfare state. Both of these elements are crucial to understanding the form taken by anti-lone mother discourse in Britain. However, there is another strand to this discourse, one that applies equally in Britain and the United States: that of anti-feminism.

The notion of 'backlash' has achieved some popular and academic credibility recently, with the publication of Susan Faludi's work about anti-feminism in the United States and Britain (Faludi 1992) and an article by Walby (1993), which add to the literature about the gender politics of the New Right and Thatcherism (e.g. ten Tusscher 1986; McNeil 1991; Somerville 1992). Both Franklin *et al.* (1991) and Walby (1993) have problematized the concept of 'backlash'. We agree with Franklin *et al.* (1991: 42) that to conceive of the gender politics of Thatcherism, or indeed any recent conservative government in Britain or the USA, as a straightforward 'backlash' against feminism is problematic, as it implies too simplistic a model of social and cultural change. Walby's (1993) critique of Faludi's analysis of the 1980s as a period of concerted effort to push women back into the home is also apposite; such a project gained less ground in Britain than in the USA. Indeed, even in the USA, women's participation in paid work continued to increase, and divorce and unmarried motherhood rates continued to climb. This said, an 'anti-feminist backlash' can be observed in discourses about lone mothers and the underclass in Britain in 1993, and in the anti-lone-mother discourse of the early 1990s in the United States; they can be seen as part of a project of 'patriarchal reconstruction' (Smart 1989).

In general, this backlash is directed against feminism and against many of the social changes of the past two decades that have reduced women's economic and social dependence on men. Walby (1990) suggests that women's increased involvement in paid work and the increase in divorce and births outside marriage are part of a shift from a private to a more public form of patriarchy (see Fox Harding,

Chapter 7 of this volume), in which women are less likely to be wholly financially dependent on a husband, and more likely to be dependent on paid work or the state. In the discourse of the backlash, however, the specificities of these social and economic changes are rarely discussed; rather blame is laid at the door of 'trendy theories' propagated by the likes of the authors and the readers of this book. For example a *Sunday Times* leader stated:

> Over the past 20 years, an assorted collection of sociologists, feminists, left wing ideologues and agony aunties have made the abnormal family into the norm.
>
> (*Sunday Times*, 11 July 1993)

A 'focus special' identified a group of American and British intellectuals – Alvin Toffler, Gloria Steinem, Germaine Greer, Harriet Harman, Neil Kinnock, Jenni Murray and Susie Orbach – as 'the pundits who made [families without men] politically correct' (*Sunday Times*, 11 July 1993).[5]

An article entitled 'The Price of Feminism' in the *Mail on Sunday* (7 March 1993) explicitly linked the murder of James Bulger with the women's liberation movement. A photograph of a 1970s march showing women carrying placards reading 'women demand equality' was placed next to a photograph of a young boy, wearing a balaclava helmet, pointing threateningly at the camera in 1993. The headline above them read 'Did this – lead to this?' In the article, Kathy Gyngell argued that feminism, by encouraging women to take paid employment, is responsible for juvenile crime and moral and social decline. Echoing theories of maternal deprivation from the 1950s (e.g. Bowlby 1951, 1953), she claimed that children were being neglected by their absent mothers, and drew upon essentialist notions of maternal instinct:

> Feminists may complain that it is unfair that mothers are primarily responsible for the upbringing of their children. But it is an unavoidable fact of life.
>     Nature provides women not only with the body to bear children, but the instinct to foster their emerging sense of morality.
>
> (*Mail on Sunday*, 7 March 1993)

The solution suggested is social policies to encourage women to stay at home with their children.

We have identified four aspects of anti-feminist backlash within recent discourses surrounding the underclass and lone motherhood.

First, there is the (re-)promotion of the heterosexual nuclear family, which Chafetz and Dworkin (1987) argue is the key feature of anti-feminist backlash. As we have shown, this is a unifying feature of recent discourses about juvenile crime, lone mothers and the underclass. Increasing rates of birth outside marriage must be halted, and fathers must return to their rightful role within the family. The degree of patriarchal power and form of paternal responsibility differs slightly between Murray's right wing and Halsey/Phillip's liberal version of the argument, but the message is the same: families need fathers. This position has been especially strong in the United States where advocates of the importance of fathers from the New Right, the fathers' rights movement and the liberal legal tradition have together created a powerful cultural force (see Fineman 1989; Brophy 1989; Smart 1989).

Second, public debates about juvenile crime and the underclass operate by reversal, in a similar way to the wider backlash (Faludi 1992; Walby 1993; Franklin et al. 1991). Thus instead of the poverty and material deprivation suffered by many lone mothers and their children being regarded as a social problem demanding policy attention, lone mothers themselves become 'the problem'. Rather than considering conditions to facilitate lone mothers being able to support their families by entering paid employment, for instance through state provision of child care, the question is how women, and men, can be powerfully dissuaded from conceiving children outside marriage (Murray 1990). Proposed solutions actually involve making life harder for lone mothers, with 'workfare', enforced sterilization, cuts in benefits and the removal of rights to social housing all being suggested.[6]

Similarly, McNeil's (1991) concept of 'the new oppressed' illustrates the way discourses over juvenile crime and the underclass operate by reversal. McNeil argues that under Thatcher a number of social groups were constructed as 'oppressed': these included parents, fathers, over-burdened taxpayers and foetuses. The rights of these groups were seen as under attack from 'female and feminist bogeys' (McNeil 1991: 229), above all, the lone mother. Thus Murray (1990), for instance, describes how difficult life is made for two-parent families who are unfortunate enough to have to try to raise their children in neighbourhoods full of single mothers and their illegitimate offspring. The decent, honest, respectable, hardworking father, the only father to attend his little girl's Christmas play, is undermined, indeed oppressed, by single mothers whose existence makes a mockery of his attempts to be a proper father.

Likewise Frank Field, a Labour MP, Chair of the Parliamentary Committee on Social Services and a noted anti-poverty campaigner, enthusiastically endorsed comments by Peter Lilley, Secretary of State for Social Security and a renowned critic of the welfare state, about the necessity of supporting 'the normal family' (Field 1993). Lilley and Field agreed that social policy should do more to support the 'traditional nurturing unit, the two-parent family', and that there was a need to reassert 'family values'. The discussion between these eminent politicians of opposite party political affiliations ended with Frank Field agreeing with Peter Lilley that previously they had 'all been too frightened to raise the issue of family values' (*Newsnight*, BBC2, 8 July 1993). Of whom these powerful men were afraid was not made explicit, but the implication was that 'political correctness' had previously prevented them from speaking their minds. This instance shows again how a myth of oppression, a reversal of actual dominant power relations, is constructed.

The third way in which discourses about juvenile crime and the underclass parallel other elements of the backlash is in its 'one-gender fixation' (Faludi 1992). Like much of the new right, these discourses are concerned primarily with the fate of young men; their attention is on the deleterious effects of unemployment for men, and of the lack of a male role model for boys. The well-being of girls and women does not enter the agenda. It could be suggested that this concern with men is an appropriate recognition that it is overwhelmingly men and boys who commit crime. However, the attention to problems of men is not the same as attention to the problem of masculinity or any sort of problematization of masculinity. On the contrary, a return to traditionally hegemonic forms of masculinity (economically dominant husband and socially dominant father) is seen as the solution to the problem. In this sense, feminist analysis and political campaigning that draw attention to the feminization of poverty and to the problems of hegemonic masculinity are implicitly attacked.

Finally, mention must be made of the essentialist constructions of masculinity and femininity that characterize much of the discourse on juvenile crime, lone mothers and the underclass. As has been pointed out earlier, Murray conceives of men and women as propelled by innate biological urges, in the case of men towards sex, and in the case of women towards procreation. These natural instincts, he argues, must be harnessed and used in a socially appropriate manner. Leaving aside the implications of social engineering, and the question of how this might be achieved, such essentialism is clearly anti-feminist.

## THE QUESTION OF AGENCY

Lurking in the shadows of this discourse about lone mothers and the underclass is an issue that we believe must be addressed head on: the issue of human agency, or in this instance, specifically, women's agency. Right-wing ideologues, conservative politicians and anti-feminists lay much of the blame for the perpetuation of the underclass through lone motherhood on the agency exercised by women; they have no trouble suggesting that women make *choices* to have children outside marriage, and without the support of a man. Defenders of lone mothers in recent debates, however, particularly the poverty lobby and feminists, have found it much harder to acknowledge women's agency.[7] In challenging the individualizing of the problems associated with lone motherhood, their focus has been on the material, structural constraints that operate on poor, working-class women. In order to refute the claims of writers such as Murray and Halsey, they seem to have thought it necessary to emphasize the lack of choices open to women with few educational qualifications in run-down inner cities. They implicitly suggest that agency is something reserved for the well-off and educated, and that while small numbers of women may be *choosing* to become lone mothers, most lone mothers are the 'victims' of their social circumstances.

This position is made explicit by Lash (1994) in his discussion of the processes of individualization and reflexive modernization that can be discerned in contemporary western societies. He criticizes the thesis advanced by Beck (1994) and Giddens (1994) that agency is progressively being freed from structure and that individuals are increasingly engaging in the reflexive construction of their own life narratives, less hindered by tradition and structure than at previous moments in history. His challenge to Beck and Giddens takes the 'single mother in the urban ghetto' as the prime exemplar of the limits of reflexive modernization:

> [J]ust how 'reflexive' is it possible for a single mother in an urban ghetto to be? Ulrich Beck and Anthony Giddens write with insight on the self-construction of life narratives. But just how much

> freedom from the 'necessity' of 'structure' and structural poverty
> does this ghetto mother have to construct her own 'life narratives'?
> (Lash 1994:120)

While we would not wish to suggest that women living in inner-city 'ghettos' can choose to escape structural poverty (but nor, probably, would Beck or Giddens), we do believe that there are women living in situations of structural poverty who are exercising agency, and consciously deciding to have children without depending on a male partner. In this sense they are undoubtedly reflexively constructing their own 'life narratives', and are not just the victims of their social circumstances. Moreover, they are not behaving very differently from middle-class unmarried women who are choosing to have children; the main difference is their poorer material circumstance. Working-class women with few educational qualifications who choose to have children outside marriage clearly make use of the meagre resources available to them to facilitate their decision: these resources include social housing and welfare benefits.

Thus we are in agreement with Beck and Beck-Gernsheim (1995) who argue that a 'new type of unmarried mother' is emerging, for whom a traditional partnership with a man is unnecessary. They cite Burkart *et al.* (1989), writing about Germany, where the rate of births outside marriage is considerably lower than in Britain or the United States:

> An illegitimate child is less and less the unwanted pregnancy of earlier years, and ever more frequently the planned pregnancy of women over 25. Extra-marital fertility, then, is less and less a 'misfortune' of young women and rather an obviously planned or at least consciously accepted decision of older women.
> (Burkart *et al.* 1989: 34, cited in Beck and Beck-Gernsheim 1995: 205)

Beck and Beck-Gernsheim acknowledge that this does not apply to a majority of women, but point to the striking change in attitudes of young women to unmarried motherhood; in 1962 89.4 per cent considered it important for a woman with a child to be married, whereas in 1983 only 40 per cent did (Allerbeck and Hoag 1985, cited in Beck and Beck-Gernsheim 1995: 205). They also point to the explosion of articles in women's magazines about lone motherhood, which not only proclaim that single mothers can be good and happy mothers, but also often offer advice on getting pregnant. There is also, they suggest, a significant theme in recent women's writing, both fiction and autobiography, which sees love for a child replacing love for a man, with the mother–child dyad replacing the cohabiting heterosexual couple as the primary source of intimacy and fulfilment in women's lives. In an individualizing society, where marriages and heterosexual partnerships are increasingly prone to failure, and where women are seeking identities for themselves, many women place trust in the permanence and stability of a relationship with a child.

We would add to Beck and Beck-Gernsheim's analysis mention of the role of feminism in this process. It is surely a measure of the success of feminism over the past century that some women have the confidence to exercise a decision to rely on the state rather than an individual man in raising their children. Probably only a small proportion of 'lone-mothers-by-choice' would identify themselves as feminists (Gordon 1990), but the creation of a cultural climate in which women are more able to live autonomous lives, is, in part, the product of the slow but deep-rooted social change that feminism has promoted.

## CONCLUSION

In this chapter we have explored the creation of a discourse that links lone mothers with the reproduction of an underclass. We have highlighted the role of the moral panic about juvenile crime in Britain in calling forth this discourse, and suggested that the perceived fiscal crisis of the welfare state and the conservative desire to reduce welfare spending have been harnessed to this discourse in both Britain and the United States. Conservative politicians in both countries, together with many liberal commentators, have reached a degree of consensus that consists of seeing the lone mother as the source of juvenile crime, welfare dependence and, ultimately, societal disintegration. The resultant call for social policy to go 'back to basics' (in Britain), or to 'restore the American dream' (in the USA) encapsulated the forlorn hope that a 'golden age' of moral turpitude, economic self-reliance and family values could be recovered. Murray's and Halsey's identification of the failure of a generation of fathers could appear to be merely a benign, if outdated, paternalism. We are less generous and it is our contention that the discourse that has developed around their work is firmly anti-feminist. Certainly in contrast to other attempts by Christian fundamentalists and moral crusaders to attach their anti-feminist campaigns to economic individualism, making use of the underclass concept has proved very successful.

This emergent consensus needs to be confronted because it constitutes an attack on feminism and, most importantly, on millions of women living in poverty. If the anti-feminism expressed by the discourse that we have analysed is to be effectively addressed and understood, we must not collude in the eradication of the agency of those who are most attacked by it. It must be recognized that lone mothers are actors in their own right and that many make active choices to be mothers.

Thus we wish to jolt the debate between right and left, anti-feminists and feminists, out of its dualisms of blame/exoneration, guilt/innocence, agent/victim. The reluctance of the poverty lobby and those sympathetic to lone mothers to address the role of agency is understandable, given the onslaught against them, but ironically it has created space for their critics. We believe that it is time to shift the agenda of the debate towards consideration of ways of enhancing the choices available to lone mothers, rather than seeking to deny them choices or to deny that they have ever exercised choice.

## NOTES

1 For a more detailed discussion of the events of 1993, see Mann and Roseneil (1994).
2 See, for example, Fox Harding (1993a, 1993b), Abbott and Wallace (1992), Solinger (1994), Spensky (1989).
3 See, for example, *Guardian*, 27 February 1993, *Sunday Times*, 28 February 1993, *The Independent*, 27 February 1993.
4 As Sinclair (1994) argues, drawing on the work of Wilensky (1975) and Sen (1981), benefits that are considered to have been 'earned', such as pensions and sickness benefit, receive far more widespread public support than those that accrue to 'the undeserving', of whom prime exemplars are non-working lone mothers.
5 For a discussion of the demonization of feminism and other liberatory movements within the academy through the construction of 'political correctness' as all powerful, see Roseneil (1995).
6 See, for example Michael Jones and Charles Murray, *Sunday Times*, 11 July 1993; Tom Sackville, Junior Health Minister, speech in Liverpool, 7 July 1993; John Redwood, Welsh Secretary, speech in Cardiff, 2 July 1993; and Michael Howard at 1993 Conservative Party Conference. See also the *Guardian*, 9 November 1993, for discussion of leaked policy document.
7 For a discussion of the poverty lobby and of the lack of attention to agency among sociologists of poverty, see Mann (1986); for a discussion of feminism's lack of attention to women's agency, see Roseneil (1995).

# References

Abbott, P. and Wallace, C. (1992) *The Family and the New Right*, London: Pluto Press.

Abramovitz, M. (1983) *Regulating the Lives of Women: The Social Functions of Public Welfare*, Boston: South End Press.

Afshar, H. (1987) 'Women, marriage and the state in Iran', in H. Afshar (ed.) *Women, State and Ideology*, London: Macmillan.

Alam, S. (1985) 'Women and poverty in Bangladesh', *Women's Studies International Forum* 8 (4): 361–71.

Alibhai-Brown, Y. (1994) 'Meet the baby fathers: men who happily have children with a handful of mothers', *Guardian*, 13 June.

Allen, J. (1983) 'Motherhood: the annihilation of women', in J. Trebilcot (ed.) *Mothering*, Savage, Md.: Rowman & Littlefield.

Allerbeck, K. and Hoag, W. (1985) *Jugend ohne Zukunft*, Munich.

Amato, P.R. (1993) 'Family structure, family process, and family ideology', *Journal of Marriage and the Family* 55: 50–54.

American Research Council (1989) *The American Family Under Siege*, Washington, DC: American Research Council.

Aries, P. (1973) *Centuries of Childhood*, Harmondsworth: Penguin.

Arshat, H. and Mohd. Yatim, M. (1989) 'The status of women in Malaysia', in K Mahadevan (ed.) *Women and Population Dynamics: Perspectives from Asian Countries*, New Dehli, London: Sage.

Babb, P. (1993) 'Teenage conceptions and fertility in England and Wales 1971–91', *Population Trends* 74 (Winter): 12–17.

Badinter, E. (1981) *The Myth of Motherhood*, London: Souvenir Press.

Bagguley, P. and Mann, K. (1992) 'Idle thieving bastards': scholarly representations of the underclass', *Work, Employment and Society* 6 (1) March: 113–26.

Banks, L. (1994) 'Angry men and working women: gender relations and economic change in Qwaqwa in the 1980s', *African Studies* 53 (1).

Barker, M. (1981) *The New Racism*, London: Junction Books.

Barrett, M. (1980) *Women's Oppression Today*, London: Verso.

Barrett, M. and McIntosh M. (1980) 'The "Family Wage": some problems for socialists and feminists', *Capital and Class* 11: 51–72.

—— (1982) *The Anti-social Family*, London: Verso.

Bart, P. (1983) 'Review of Chodorow's *The Reproduction of Mothering*', in J. Trebilcot (ed.) *Mothering*, Savage, Md.: Rowman & Littlefield.

Bartholomew, R., Hibbert, A. and Sidaway, J. (1992) 'Lone parents and the labour market: evidence from the Labour Force Survey', *Employment Gazette*, November: 559–78.

Beck, U. (1994) 'The reinvention of politics: towards a theory of reflexive modernization', in U. Beck, A. Giddens, S. Lash, *Reflexive Modernization: Politics, Tradition and Aesthetics in the Modern Social Order*, Cambridge: Polity Press.

Beck, U. and Beck-Gernsheim, E. (1995) *The Normal Chaos of Love*, Cambridge: Polity Press.

Bell, L. and Ribbens, J. (1994) 'Isolated housewives and complex maternal worlds. The significance of social contacts between women with young children in industrial societies', *Sociological Review* 42 (2): 227–62.

Berger, I. (1992) *Threads of Solidarity, Women in South African Industry 1900–1980*, London: James Currey.

Besson, J. (1993) 'Reputation and respectability reconsidered: a new perspective on Afro-Caribbean peasant women', in J.H. Momsen (ed.) *Women and Change in the Caribbean*, Kingston, Jamaica: Ian Randle; London: James Currey.

Beveridge, W. (1942) *Social Insurance and Allied Services*, London: HMSO, Cmnd 6404.

Bharat, S. (1986) 'Single-parent family in India: issues and implications', *Indian Journal of Social Work* 47 (1): 55–65.

Billig, M. (1991) *Ideology and Opinion*, London: Sage.

Björnberg, U. (1992) 'Tvåforsörjarefamiljen i teori och verklighet', in J. Acker (ed.) *Kvinnors och Mans Liv och Arbete*, Stockholm: S.N.S.

Blackie, A. (1994) 'Family fall-out', *Times Higher Education Supplement*, 4 March: 18.

Blaikie, A. (1994) 'Constructing and reconstructing sexuality in Victorian Scotland: the case of illegitimacy', paper presented to the British Sociological Association Annual Conference, Preston.

Bland, L. (1986) 'Marriage laid bare: middle-class women and marital sex, 1880–1914', in J. Lewis (ed.) *Labour and Love: Women's Experience of Home and Family, 1850–1940*, Oxford: Basil Blackwell.

Block, R. (1978) 'American feminine ideals in transition: the rise of the moral mother, 1785–1815', *Feminist Studies* 4 (2): 101–26.

Boris, E. (1989) 'Homework and women's rights: the case of the Vermont knitters: 1980–85', in E. Boris and C. Daniels (eds) *Homework. Historical and Contemporary Perspectives on Paid Labor at Home*, Urbana and Chicago: University of Illinois Press.

Bowlby, J. (1946) *Forty-four Juvenile Thieves: Their Characters and Home-life*, London: Bailliere, Tindall & Cox (first published 1944, *International Journal of Psycho-analysis* XXV: 55–6).

—— (1951) *Maternal Care and Mental Health*, Geneva: World Health Organization.

—— (1953) *Child Care and the Growth of Love*, Harmondsworth: Penguin.

Bozzoli, B. (1983) 'Marxism, feminism and South African studies', *Journal of Southern African Studies* 9 (2): 139–71.

Bradshaw, J. (1989) *Lone Parents: Policy in the Doldrums*, London: Family Policy Studies Centre.
Bradshaw, J. and Millar, J. (1991) *Lone Parent Families in the UK*, London: HMSO.
Bradshaw, J., Ditch, J., Holmes, H. and Whiteford, P. (1993) *Support for Children: A Comparison of the Arrangements in Fifteen Countries*, London: HMSO.
Brah, A. (1993) 'Re-framing Europe: en-gendered racisms, ethnicities and nationalisms in contemporary western Europe', *Feminist Review* 45: 9–28.
Brannen, J. and Moss, P. (1991) *Managing Mothers: Dual Earner Households after Maternity Leave*, London: Unwin Hyman.
Braverman, H. (1974) *Labor and Monopoly Capital: The Degradation of Work in the Twentieth Century*, London: Monthly Review Press.
Brindle, D. (1995a) 'Right group says Tories anti-family', *Guardian*, 3 January 1995.
—— (1995b) 'Lilley targets 1.4bn pounds benefit fraud', *Guardian*, 11 July 1995,
Brittan, A. and Maynard, M. (1984) *Sexism, Racism and Oppression*, Oxford: Basil Blackwell.
Brocas, A-M., Cailloux, A-M. and Oget, V. (1990) *Women and Social Security: Progress Towards Equality of Treatment*, Geneva: International Labour Organisation.
Brookes, B. (1986) 'Women and reproduction, 1860–1939', in J. Lewis (ed.) *Labour and Love: Women's Experience of Home and Family, 1850–1940*, Oxford: Basil Blackwell.
Brophy, J. (1989) 'Custody law, child care and inequality in Britain', in C. Smart and S. Sevenhuijsen (eds) *Child Custody and the Politics of Gender*, London: Routledge.
Brown, C. (1981) 'Mothers, fathers and children: from private to public patriarchy', in L. Sargent (ed.) *Women and Revolution: The Unhappy Marriage of Marxism and Feminism*, London: Pluto Press.
Brown, J. (1989) *Why Don't They Go to Work? Mothers on Benefit*, London: HMSO.
Brown, M. (1995) 'Demographic trends', in L. Burghes, *Single Lone Parents. Problems, Prospects and Policies*, London, Family Policy Studies Centre.
Bruegel, I. (1989) 'Sex and race in the labour market', *Feminist Review* 32: 49–68.
Buchanan, E. (1994) 'Bogota death squads dispose of the poor', *Independent on Sunday*, 30 January.
Buck, N., Gershuny, J., Rose, D. and Scott, J. (eds) (1994) *Changing Households: The British Household Panel Survey 1990–1992*, ESRC Centre on Micro-social Change, Colchester: University of Essex.
Bunting, M. (1994) 'Get the poor off our over-taxed backs', interview with Charles Murray, *Guardian*, 17 September.
Burawoy, M. (1985) *The Politics of Production: Factory Regimes Under Capitalism and Socialism*, London: Verso.
Burghes, L. (1993) *One-Parent Families: Policy Options for the 1990s*, York: Family Policy Studies Centre/Joseph Rowntree Foundation.

214    References

—— (1994) *Lone Parenthood and Family Disruption: The Outcomes for Children*, London: Family Policy Studies Centre.

Burgoyne, C. and Millar, J. (1994) 'Enforcing child support obligations: the views of separated fathers', *Policy and Politics* 22 (2): 95–104.

Burkart, G., Fietze, B. and Kohli, M. (1989) *Liebe, Ehe, Elternschaft*, Materialen zur Bevolkerungswissenschaft, No. 60, Wiesbaden: Bundesinstitut für Bevolkerungsforschung.

Burns, A. and Scott, C. (1994) *Mother-Headed Families and Why They Have Increased*, Hillsdale, NJ: Lawrence Erlbaum Associates.

Bussemaker, J. and van Kersbergen, K. (1994) 'Gender and welfare states: some theoretical reflections', in D. Sainsbury (ed.) *Gendering Welfare States*, London: Sage.

Butler, J. (1990) *Gender Trouble*, London: Routledge.

Buvinic, M., Valenzuela, J.P., Molina, T. and González, E. (1992) 'The fortunes of adolescent mothers and their children: a case study on the transmission of poverty in Santiago, Chile', *Population and Development Review* 18 (2): 269–97.

Cain, M. (1982) 'Perspectives on family and fertility in developing countries', *Population Studies* 36 (2): 159–76.

Caldwell, J. (1982) *The Theory of Fertility Decline*, New York: Academic Press.

Capaldi, D.M. (1992) 'Step-families: an American perspective', *Family Policy Bulletin*, June, London: Family Policy Studies Centre.

Capaldi, D.M and Patterson, G.R (1991), 'Relation of parental transitions to boys' adjustment problems', *Developmental Psychology* 27 (33): 489–504.

Carling, A. (1991) *Social Divisions*, London: Verso.

Cass, B. (1992) 'Caring work and welfare regimes: policies for sole parents in four countries', in S. Shaver (ed.) *Comparative Perspectives on Sole Parent Policy: Work and Welfare*, Proceedings of a seminar, University of New South Wales: Social Policy Research Centre.

Caunce, S. and Honeyman, K. (1993) 'Introduction: the city of Leeds and its business 1893–1993', in J. Chartres and K. Honeyman (eds) *Leeds City Business*, Centre for Business History, Leeds: Leeds University Press.

Chafetz, J.S. and Dworkin, A.G. (1987) 'In the face of threat: organised antifeminism in comparative perspective', *Gender and Society* 1 (1): 33–60.

Chandler, J. (1991) *Women Without Husbands: An Exploration of the Margins of Marriage*, London: Macmillan.

Chant, S. (1991) *Women and Survival in Mexican Cities: Perspectives on Gender, Labour Markets and Low-Income Households*, Manchester: Manchester University Press.

Chase-Lansdale, P.L. and Hetherington, E.M. (1990) 'The impact of divorce on life-span development: short and long-term effects', in P.B. Baltes, D.L. Featherman and R.M. Lerner (eds) *Life-Span Development and Behaviour*, Volume 10, Hillsdale, NH: Lawrence Erlbaum Associates.

Cherlin, A.J., Furstenburg, F.F., Chase-Lansdale, P.L., Kiernan, K.E., Robins, P.K., Morrison, D.R. and Teieler, J.O. (1991) 'Longitudinal studies of effects of divorce on children in Great Britain and the United States', *Science* 252 (June): 1386–9.

Child Poverty Action Group (1990) *The Poverty of Maintenance, A Response*

*From the Child Poverty Action Group to the White Paper on Maintenance, Children Come First*, London: Child Poverty Action Group.

—— (1993a) Press release *Child Support Handbook Published as new Child Maintenance Scheme Comes Under Attack*, 6 April 1993, London: Child Poverty Action Group.

—— (1993b) 'Child support', *Poverty* 85: 2–3.

Child Support Evaluation Advisory Group (1992) *Child Support in Australia*. Final report of the evaluation, vols 1 and 2, Canberra: Commonwealth of Australia.

Clark, A. (1919) *Working Life of Women in the Seventeenth Century*, London: Routledge & Kegan Paul (reprinted 1982).

Clark, A. (1992) 'The rhetoric of Chartist domesticity: gender, language, and class in the 1830s and 1840s', *Journal of British Studies* 31: 62–88.

Clarke, J., Cochrane, A. and Smart, C. (1987) *Ideologies of Welfare*, London: Hutchinson.

Clarke, K., Glendinning, C. and Craig, G. (1994a) 'Down the drain', Community Care, 29 September–9 October 1994.

—— (1994b) *Losing Support: Children and the Child Support Act*, London: The Children's Society.

Cochran, M., Larner, M., Riley, D., Gunnarsson, L. and Henderson, C.R. (1993) *Extending Families: The Social Networks of Parents and Their Children*, Cambridge: Cambridge University Press.

Cock, J. (1980) *Maids and Madams: A Study in the Politics of Exploitation*, Johannesburg: Raven Press.

Cockett, M. and Tripp, J. (1994) *Family Breakdown and its Impact on Children: The Exeter Study*, England, University of Exeter Press.

Cohen, B. and Fraser, N. (1991) *Childcare in a Modern Welfare State*, London: Institute for Public Policy Research.

Commission for Racial Equality (1984) *Report of an Investigation into Racial Discrimination in Housing*, London: Commission for Racial Equality.

*Community Care*, brief articles on the following dates: 7 March 1991; 13 June 1991; 9 September 1991; 21 October 1991; 11 November 1991; 16/23 December 1991; 7 May 1994.

Cotterill, P. (1994) *Friendly Relations? Mothers and Their Daughters-in-Law*, London: Taylor & Francis.

Cousins, C. (1994) 'A comparison of the labour market position of women in Spain and the UK with reference to the "flexible" labour debate', *Work, Employment and Society* 8 (1): 45–67.

Cowan, R. (1983) *More Work for Mother: The Ironies of Household Technology from the Open Hearth to the Microwave*, New York: Basic Books.

Cretney, S. (1987) *Elements of Family Law*, London: Sweet & Maxwell.

Crow, G. and Hardey, M. (1992) 'Diversity and ambiguity among lone-parent households in modern Britain', in C. Marsh and S. Arber (eds) *Families and Households: Divisions and Change*, Basingstoke: Macmillan.

Dagenais, H. (1993) 'Women in Guadeloupe: the Paradoxes of Reality', in J.H. Momsen (ed.) *Women and Change in the Caribbean*, Kingston, Jamaica: Ian Randle; London: James Currey.

Davidoff, L. (1979) 'The separation of home and work? Landladies and

lodgers in nineteenth and twentieth century England', in S. Burman (ed.) *Fit Work for Women*, London: Croom Helm.
—— (1995) *Worlds Between: Historical Perspectives on Gender and Class*, Cambridge: Polity Press.
Davidoff, L. and Hall, C. (1987) *Family Fortunes: Men and Women of the English Middle Class 1780–1850*, London: Hutchinson.
Davies, J. (ed.) (1993) *The Family: Is It Just Another Lifestyle Choice?*, London: Institute of Economic Affairs, Health and Welfare Unit.
Davin, A. (1978) 'Imperialism and motherhood', *History Workshop Journal* 5: 19–65.
Dean, H. and Taylor-Gooby, P. (1992) *Dependency Culture*, Hemel Hempstead: Harvester Wheatsheaf.
Demo, D.H. (1993) 'The relentless search for effects of divorce: forging new trails or tumbling down the beaten path', *Journal of Marriage and the Family* 55: 42–5.
Dennis, N. and Erdos, G. (1992) *Families without Fatherhood*, London: Institute of Economic Affairs, Health and Welfare Unit (2nd edn 1993).
Department of Social Security (1991) *The Government's Expenditure Plans 1991–92 to 1993–94*, Cm. 1514, London: HMSO.
—— (1993a) *The Growth of Social Security*, London, HMSO.
—— (1993b) *Child Support Act: Secretary of State Guidelines on the Application of the Requirement to Co-operate*, London: HMSO.
—— (1995) *Improving Child Support*, London: HMSO.
Dickerson, B. (ed) (1995) *African American Single Mothers: Understanding their Lives and Families*, London: Sage.
Dilnot, A. and Duncan, A. (1992) 'Lone mothers, family credit and paid work', *Fiscal Studies* 13: 1.
Donzelot, J. (1979) *The Policing of Families*, London: Hutchinson.
Duncan, S. (1991a) 'The geography of gender divisions of labour in Britain', *Transactions*, Institute of British Geographers, NS, 16: 420–39.
—— (1991b) 'Gender divisions of labour', in D. Green and K. Hoggart (eds) *London: A New Metropolitan Geography*, London: Allen & Unwin.
—— (1994) 'Theorising differences in patriarchy', *Environment and Planning* 26 (8): 1177–94.
—— (1996) 'The diverse worlds of European patriarchy', in D.M. García-Ramon and J. Monk (eds) *Women of the European Union: The Politics of Work and Daily Life*, London: Routledge.
Duncan, S. and Edwards, R. (1997, forthcoming) *Lone Mothers and Paid Work: Context, Discourse and Action*, London: Macmillan.
Duza, A. (1989) 'Bangladesh women in transition: dynamics and issues', in K. Mahadevan (ed.) *Women and Population Dynamics: Perspectives from Asian Countries*, New Dehli, London: Sage.
Dwyer, D. and Bruce, J. (eds) (1988) *A Home Divided: Women and Income in the Third World*, Stanford, Calif.: Stanford University Press.
Edholm, F. (1982) 'The unnatural family', in E. Whitelegg *et al.* (eds) *The Changing Experience of Women*, Oxford: Blackwell
Edwards, J., Fuller, T., Vorakitphokatoru, S. and Sermsri, S. (1992) 'Female employment and marital instability: evidence from Thailand', *Journal of Marriage and the Family* 54 (1): 59–68.

Edwards, R. (1992) 'Evaluation of the Department of Health's new Under Fives Initiative lone parents projects', London: National Children's Bureau.

——(1993) 'Taking the initiative: the government, lone mothers and day care provision', *Critical Social Policy* 39: 36–50.

Edwards, R. and Duncan, S. (1996) 'Lone mothers and economic activity', in F. Williams (ed.) *Social Policy: A Critical Reader*, Cambridge: Polity Press.

Edwards, R. and Ribbens, J. (1991) ' "Meanderings around strategy": a research note on strategic discourse in the lives of women', *Sociology* 25 (3): 477–90.

Edwards, S. and Halpern, A. (1992) 'Parental responsibility: an instrument of social policy', *Family Law* 22: 113–18.

Eekelaar, J. (1991) 'Parental responsiblity: state of nature or nature of the state?, *Journal of Social Welfare and Family Law* 1: 37–50.

Ehrenreich, B. (1983) *The Hearts of Men: American Dreams and the Flight from Commitment*, London: Pluto Press.

Ehrenreich, B. and English, D. (1979) *For Her Own Good: 150 Years of the Experts' Advice to Women*, London: Pluto Press.

Elliott, B.J. (1991) 'Demographic trends in domestic life', in D. Clark (ed.) *Marriage, Domestic Life and Social Change. Writings for Jacqueline Burgoyne 1944–88*, London: Routledge.

Elliott, B.J. and Richards, M.P.M. (1991) 'Children and divorce: educational performance and behaviour before and after parental separation', *International Journal of Law and the Family* 5 (3): 258–76.

Ellis, K. (1981) 'Can the Left defend a fantasized family?', *In These Times*, 9 December.

Epstein, T.S., Crehan, K., Gerzer, A. and Sass, J. (1986) *Women, Work and Family in Britain and Germany*, London: Croom Helm.

Ermisch, J. (1986) *The Economics of the Family: Applications to Divorce and Re-marriage*, London: Centre for Economic Policy Research.

——(1991) *Lone Parents: An Economic Analysis*, Cambridge: Cambridge University Press.

Ermisch, J. and Wright, R. (1991) 'Welfare benefits and lone parents' employment in the UK', *Journal of Human Resources* 26: 829–44.

Esping-Andersen, G. (1990) *The Three Worlds of Welfare Capitalism*, Cambridge: Polity Press.

Etzioni, A. (1994) *The Spirit of Community: Rights, Responsibilities and the Communitarian Agenda*, New York: Simon & Schuster.

Everingham, C. (1994) *Motherhood and Modernity: An Investigation into the Rational Dimension of Mothering*, Buckingham: Open University Press.

Faludi, S. (1992) *Backlash: The Undeclared War against Women*, London: Chatto & Windus.

Farrington, D. (1994) 'The influence of the family on delinquent development', in C. Henricson (ed.) *Crime and the Family: Conference Report*, London: Family Policy Studies Centre.

Ferguson, A. (1983) 'On conceiving motherhood and sexuality: a feminist materialist approach', in J. Trebilcot (ed.) *Mothering*, Savage, Md.: Rowman & Littlefield.

Ferguson, A. (1989) *Blood at the Root: Motherhood, Sexuality and Male Dominance*, London: Pandora Press.

Ferri, E. (1976) *Growing Up in a One-Parent Family*, Windsor: National Foundation for Education Research–Nelson.

Field, F. (1993) 'Fairness for two-family fathers', *Guardian*, 27 October 1993.

Fildes, V. (1988) *Wet Nursing: a History from Antiquity to the Present*, Oxford: Basil Blackwell.

Finch, J. (1994) 'Families, generations and policy relevant research', paper presented to the annual conference of the Social Policy Association, University of Liverpool.

Fineman, M. (1989) 'The politics of custody and gender: child advocacy and the transformation of custody decision making in the USA', in C. Smart and S. Sevenhuijsen (eds) *Child Custody and the Politics of Gender*, London: Routledge.

Finer, M. (1974) *Report of the Committee on One Parent Families*, London: HMSO, Cmnd 5629.

Flandrin, J.L. (1979) *Families in Former Times*, Cambridge: Cambridge University Press

Flowerdew, R. and Green, A. (1993) 'Migration, transport and workplace statistics from the 1991 census', in A. Dale and C. Marsh (eds) *The 1991 Census Users' Guide*, London: HMSO.

Folbre, N. (1983) 'Of patriarchy born: the political economy of fertility decisions', Feminist Studies 9 (2): 261–84.

—— (1986) 'Cleaning house: new perspectives on households and economic development', *Journal of Development Economics* 22: 5–40.

—— (1991) *Mothers on Their Own: Policy Issues for Developing Countries*, New York: Population Council.

—— (1994) *Who Pays For The Kids?: Gender and the Structures of Constraint*, London: Routledge.

Forna, M. (1995) 'The myth and the mister', *Guardian*, 21 March 1995.

Foucault, M. (1972) *The Archaeology of Knowledge*, London: Tavistock.

—— (1980) *Power/Knowledge*, Brighton: Harvester.

—— (1981) *The History of Sexuality*, Vol. 1: *An Introduction*, Harmondsworth: Penguin.

Fox Harding, L. (1993a) 'Alarm versus Liberation? Responses to the increase in lone parents – Part 1', *The Journal of Social Welfare and Family Law* 2: 101–12.

—— (1993b) 'Alarm versus Liberation? Responses to the increase in lone parents – Part 2', *The Journal of Social Welfare and Family Law* 3: 174–84.

—— (1994) 'Parental responsibility: a dominant theme in British child and family policy for the 1990s', *International Journal of Sociology and Social Policy* 14 (1/2): 84–105.

Franklin, S., Lury, C. and Stacey, J. (eds) (1991) *Off-Centre: Feminism and Cultural Studies*, London: Harper Collins.

Friedan, B. (1963) *The Feminine Mystique*, London: Penguin.

Furstenberg, F., Brooks-Gunn, J. and Morgan, S.P. (1987) *Adolescent Mothers in Later Life*, Cambridge: Cambridge University Press.

Furstenberg, F.F. Jr. and Cherlin, A.J. (1991) *Divided Families: What Happens to Children When Parents Part?*, Cambridge, Mass.: Harvard University Press.

Gardiner, J. (1996) *Gender, Care and the Economy*, Basingstoke: Macmillan.

Garfinkel, I. and Wong, Y. (1990) 'Child support and public policy', in *Lone Parents: The Economic Challenge*, Paris: Organization for Economic Co-operation and Development.

Garnham, A. (1993) Newspoints, 'Child Support Act may lead to increase in adoption', *Adoption and Fostering* 17 (2): 2–3.

Garnham, A. and Knights, E. (1994) *Putting the Treasury First: The Truth About Child Support*, London: Child Poverty Action Group.

Geisler, G., Keller, B. and Chuzu, P. (1985), *The Needs of Rural Women in Northern Province: Analysis and Recommendations*, a report prepared for NCDP and NORAD, Lusaka: GRZ Printer.

Gershuny, J. and Brice, J. (1994) 'Looking backwards: family and work 1900 to 1992', in N. Buck, J. Gershuny, D. Rose, and J. Scott (eds) *Changing Households*, ESRC Research Centre, Colchester: University of Essex.

GHS (1994), *General Household Survey 1992*, London: HMSO.

Giddens, A. (1992) *The Transformation of Intimacy*, Cambridge: Polity Press.

—— (1994) 'Living in a post-traditional society', in U. Beck, A. Giddens and S. Lash (eds) *Reflexive Modernization: Politics, Tradition and Aesthetics in the Modern Social Order*, Cambridge: Polity Press.

Giles, J. (1995) *Women, Identity and Private Life in Britain, 1900–50*, Basingstoke: Macmillan.

Gillis, J. (1979) 'Servants, sexual relations, and the risks of illegitimacy in London, 1801– 1900', *Feminist Studies* 5 (1): 142–73.

Gilroy, P. (1987) *There Ain't No Black in the Union Jack*, London: Hutchinson.

Glenn, E.N., Chang, G. and Forcey, L.R. (eds) (1994) *Mothering. Ideology, Experience and Agency*, London: Routledge.

Glucksmann, M. (1990) *Women Assemble: Women Workers and the New Industries in the Inter-war Britain*. London: Routledge.

Goode, W.J. (1963) *World Revolution and Family Patterns*, New York: Collier Macmillan.

Goode, W. (1993) *World Changes in Divorce Patterns*, New Haven and London: Yale University Press.

Gordon, T. (1990) *Feminist Mothers*, London: Macmillan.

—— (1994) *Single Women*, London: Macmillan.

Government of the Republic of Zambia, CSO (1993) *Social Dimensions of Adjustment, Priority Survey I, 1991*, Lusaka: Government Printer.

Green, D. (1993) 'Foreword', in J. Davies (ed.) *The Family: Is it Just Another Lifestyle Choice?* London: Institute of Economic Affairs, Health and Welfare Unit.

Gregson, N. and Lowe, M. (1994) *Servicing the Middle Classes: Class, Gender and Waged Domestic Labour in Contemporary Britain*, London: Routledge.

Griffin, C. (1993) *Representations of Youth*, Cambridge: Polity Press.

Gustafsson, S. (1990) 'Labour force participation and the earnings of lone parents: a Swedish case study including comparisons with Germany', in *Lone parents: the economic challenge*, Paris: Organisation for Economic Co-operation and Development.

Gustafsson, B. and Kjulin, U. (1992) *'Barnomsorg och hushallsarbete'*, Forskaresyposium, Sigtuna.

Gustafsson, B. and Klevmarken, N.A. (1994) 'Taxes and transfers in Sweden: incentive effects on labour supply', in A.B. Atkinson and G.V. Mogensen (eds) *Welfare and Work Incentives: A North European Perspective*, Oxford: Clarendon Press.

Haaga, J. and Mason, J. (1987) 'Food distribution within the family: evidence and implications for research and programs', *Food Policy* (May): 146–60.

Hakim, C. (1993) 'The myth of the rising female employment', *Work, Employment and Society* 7 (1): 97–120.

—— (1994) 'A century of change in occupational segregation 1881–1991', *Journal of Historical Sociology* 7 (4): 435–54.

Hall, C. (1979) 'The early formation of Victorian domestic ideology', in S. Burman (ed.) *Fit Work for Women*, London: Croom Helm.

—— (1980) 'The history of the housewife', in E. Mallos (ed.) *The Politics of Housework*, London: Allison & Busby.

Hall, S. (1992) 'The West and the rest: discourse and power', in S. Hall and B. Gieben (eds) *Formations of Modernity*, Cambridge: Polity Press.

Hall, S., Critcher, C., Jefferson, T., Clarke, J. and Roberts, B. (1978) *Policing the Crisis: Mugging, the State and Law and Order*, Basingstoke: Macmillan.

Halsey, A.H. (1991) 'Time to rebuild the traditional family', *Financial Times*, 12 August.

——(1992) Foreword to N. Dennis and G. Erdos, *Families without Fatherhood* London: Institute of Economic Affairs, Health and Welfare Unit, Choice in Welfare No. 12.

Hansen, K. (1989) *Distant Companions: Servants and Employers in Zambia, 1900–1985*, Ithaca, NY: Cornell University Press.

—— (ed.) (1992) *African Encounters with Domesticity*, New Brunswick, NJ: Rutgers University Press.

Hardey, M. and Crow, G. (eds) (1991) *Lone Parenthood: Coping with Constraints and Making Opportunities*, London: Harvester Wheatsheaf.

Haskey, J. (1990) 'Children in families broken by divorce', *Population Trends* 61 (Autumn): 34–42.

—— (1993) 'First marriage, divorce and remarriage: birth cohort analysis', *Population Trends* 72 (Summer): 24–33.

—— (1994) 'Estimated numbers of one-parent families and their prevalence in Great Britain in 1991', *Population Trends* 78 (Winter): 5–19.

Heath, S and Dale, A (1994) 'Household and family formation in Great Britain: the ethnic dimension', *Population Trends* 77 (Autumn): 5–13.

Held, V. (1983) 'The obligations of mothers and fathers', in J. Trebilcot (ed.) *Mothering*, Savage, Md.: Rowman & Littlefield.

Hewitt, P. and Leach, P. (1993) *Social Justice, Children and Families*, London: Institute for Public Policy and Research.

Hirdmann, Y. (1990) 'Genussystemet', in *Statens Offentliga Utredningar*, Demokrati och Makt i Sverige, SOU 1990: 44.

Hobson, B. (1994) 'Sole mothers, social policy regimes and the logics of gender', in Sainsbury, D. (ed.) *Gendering Welfare States*, London: Sage.

Hodgson, G. (1988) *Economic Institutions*, Cambridge: Polity Press.

Hollis, M. and Nell, E. (1975) *Rational Economic Man: A Philosophical Critique of Neo-classical Economics*, London: Cambridge University Press.

Holtermann, S. (1992) *Investing in Young Children: Costing an Education and Day Care Service*, London: National Children's Bureau.

Horn, P. (1990) *The Rise and Fall of the Victorian Servant*, Stroud, Gloucestershire: Alan Sutton (1st edn 1975).

Humphries, J. (1987) ' "... The most free from objection ..." : the sexual division of labor and women's work in nineteenth-century England', *Journal of Economic History* XLVII (4): 929–49.

Humphries, S. and Gordon, P. (1993) *A Labour of Love. The Experience of Parenthood in Britain 1900–1950*, London: Sidgwick & Jackson.

International Year of the Family (1994) *Parents and Families*, Factsheet 5, available from the Family Policy Studies Centre, London.

James, A. and Prout, A. (eds) (1990) *Constructing and Reconstructing Childhood*, Brighton: Falmer Press.

Jazairy, I., Alamgir, M. and Panuccio, T. (1992) *The State of World Rural Poverty, an Inquiry into its Causes and Consequences*, London: IT Publications.

Jenkins, S. (1992) 'Lone mothers' employment and full-time work possibilities', *Economic Journal*, March: 310–20.

Jolly, M. and Macintyre, M. (eds) (1989) *Family and Gender in the Pacific*, Cambridge: Cambridge University Press.

Jordan, B., Simon, J., Kay, H. and Redley, M. (1992) *Trapped in Poverty: Labour Market Decisions in Low-Income Households*, London: Routledge.

Joshi, H. (ed.) (1989) *The Changing Population of Britain*, Oxford: Blackwell.

Kahn, A.J. and Kamerman, S.B. (1983) *Income Transfers for Families with Children*, Philadelphia: Temple University Press.

—— (1988) *Child Support*, New York: Sage.

Kaplan, E.A. (1992) *Motherhood and Representation*, London: Routledge.

Keith, M. (1993) *Race, Riots and Policing: Lore and Disorder in a Multi-racist Society*, London: UCL Press.

Kennedy, E. (1992) 'Effects of gender of head of household on women's and children's nutritional status', paper presented at the workshop on The Effects of Policies and Programs on Women, 16 January 1992, Washington, DC.

Kiernan, K. (1992a) 'The impact of family disruption in childhood on transitions made in young adult life', *ESRC Data Archive Bulletin*, Colchester: University of Essex.

—— (1992b) 'The impact of family disruption in childhood on transitions made in young adult life', *Population Studies* 46: 213–34.

Kiernan, K. and Wicks, M. (1990) *Family Change and Future Policy*, York: Family Policy Studies Centre/Joseph Rowntree Memorial Trust.

Kinsey, R. (1993) 'Innocent underclass', *New Statesman and Society*, 5 March: 16–17.

Kittay, E. (1983) 'Womb envy: an explanatory concept', in J. Trebilcot, *Mothering*, Savage, Md.: Rowman & Littlefield.

Kuh, D. and Maclean, M. (1990) 'Women's childhood experience of parental separation and their subsequent health and status in adulthood', *Journal of Biosocial Science* 22: 121–35.

Land, H. (1980) 'The family wage', *Feminist Review* 6: 55–76.
—— (1993) 'The demise of the male breadwinner in practice but not in theory: a challenge for social security systems', in S. Baldwin and J. Falkingham (eds) *Social Security and Social Change*, London: Simon & Schuster.

Laqueur, T. (1990) *Making Sex*, Cambridge, Mass.: Harvard University Press.

Lasch, C. (1977) *Haven in a Heartless World: The Family Beseiged*, New York: W.W. Norton.

Lash, S. (1994) 'Reflexivity and its doubles: structure, aesthetics, community', in U. Beck, A. Giddens, S. Lash (eds) *Reflexive Modernization: Politics, Tradition and Aesthetics in the Modern Social Order*, Cambridge: Polity Press.

Laslett, P. (1977) *Family Life and Illicit Love in Earlier Generations*, Cambridge: Cambridge University Press.

Lauras-Lecoh, T. (1990) 'Family trends and demographic transition in Africa', *International Social Science Journal* 42: 475–92.

Lawrence, E. (1982) 'In the abundance of water the fool is thirsty: sociology and black "pathology" ', in Centre for Contemporary Cultural Studies (ed.) *The Empire Strikes Back: Race and Racism in 70s Britain*, London: Hutchinson.

Leira, A. (1992) *Welfare States and Working Mothers*, Cambridge: Cambridge University Press.

Lewis, J. (1984) *Women in England 1870–1950: Sexual Divisions and Social Change*, Hemel Hempstead: Harvester Wheatsheaf.
—— (ed.) (1986) *Labour and Love: Women's Experience of Home and Family, 1850–1940*, Oxford: Basil Blackwell.
—— (1989) 'Lone parent families: politics and economics', *Journal of Social Policy* 18 (4): 595–600.
—— (1992a) *Women in Britain since 1945: Women, Family, Work and the State in the Post-war Years*, Oxford: Basil Blackwell.
—— (1992b) 'Gender and the development of welfare regimes', *Journal of European Social Policy* 2 (3): 159–73.

Liddiard, M (1923) *The Mothercraft Manual*, London: Churchill.

Lister, R. (1994) 'The Child Support Act; shifting family financial obligations in the UK', *Social Politics* 1 (2): 211–22.

Lloyd, C. and Gage-Brandon, A. (1993) 'Women's role in maintaining households: family welfare and sexual inequality in Ghana', *Population Studies* 47: 115–31.

'London Women's Liberation Campaign for Legal and Financial Independence' and 'Rights of Women' (1979) 'Disaggregation now! Another battle for women's independence', *Feminist Review*, Number 2: 19–31.

Lord Chancellor, Secretary of State for Scotland, Secretary of State for Social Security, Secretary of State for Northern Ireland, Lord Advocate (1990) *Children Come First: The Government's Proposals on the Maintenance of Children*, Cm. 1264, London: HMSO.

Lorenzo, R. (1993) *Italy: Too Little Time and Space for Childhood*, Florence: Innocenti Report, Unicef.

McAdoo, H.P. (1988) *Black Families: Second Edition*, Newbury, California: Sage.

McCashin, A. (1993) *Lone Parents in the Republic of Ireland*, Dublin: The Economic and Social Research Institute.

McGlone, F. (1994) 'From back to basics to common ground', *Family Policy Bulletin*, December, London: Family Policy Studies Centre.

MacGregor, S. (1990) 'Could Britain inherit the American nightmare?', in *British Journal of Addiction* 85 (7): 863–72.

McIntyre, S. (1976) ' "Who wants babies?" The social construction of "instincts" ', in D. Leonard Barker and S. Allen (eds) *Sexual Divisions and Society*, London: Tavistock.

Mckay, S. and Marsh, A. (1994) *Lone Parenthood and Work*, Research Report No. 25, Department of Social Security, London: HMSO.

McKendrick, J. (n.d.) 'Lone parenthood in the nineties', School of Geography, University of Manchester.

McLagan, I. (1992) *A Broken Promise: The Failure of Youth Training Policy*, London: Youthaid and the Children's Society.

McLanahan, S. (1988) 'The consequences of single parenthood for subsequent generations', *Focus* 11 (3): 16–21, Institute for Research on Poverty, University of Wisconsin-Madison.

McLanahan, S. and Bumpass, I. (1988) 'Intergenerational consequences of family disruption', *American Journal of Sociology* 94· 130–52.

McLaren, A. (1992) *A History of Contraception*, Oxford: Blackwell.

Maclean, M. and Wadsworth, M.E.J. (1988) 'The interest of children after parental divorce: a long-term perspective', *International Journal of Law and the Family*:155–66.

McNeil, M. (1991) 'Making and not making the difference: the gender politics of Thatcherism', in S. Franklin, C. Lury and J. Stacey (eds) *Off-Centre: Feminism and Cultural Studies*, London: Harper Collins.

Macnicol, J. (1987) 'In pursuit of the underclass', *Journal of Social Policy* 16 (3): 293–318.

Macnicol, L. (1980) *The Movement for Family Allowances, 1918–45*, London: Heinemann.

McRae, S. (1993) *Cohabiting Mothers: Changing Marriage and Motherhood?*, London: Policy Studies Institute.

McRobbie, A. (1989) *From Jackie to Just Seventeen*, London: Macmillan.

Mädje, E. and Neusüss, C. (1994) 'Lone mothers in Berlin: disadvantaged citizens or women escaping patriarchy', *The Diverse Worlds of European Patriarchy: Environment and Planning* 26A (9): 1419 33.

Mann, K. (1986) 'The making of a claiming class: the neglect of agency in analyses of the welfare state', *Critical Social Policy* 15 (Spring): 62–74.

—— (1992) *The Making of an English 'Underclass'? The Social Divisions of Welfare and Labour*, Buckingham: Open University Press.

Mann, K. and Roseneil, S. (1994) ' "Some Mothers Do 'Ave 'Em": backlash and the gender politics of the underclass debate', *Journal of Gender Studies* 3 (3): 317–31.

Mark-Lawson, J. (1988) 'Occupational segregation and women's politics', in S. Walby (ed.) *Gender Segregation at Work*, Milton Keynes: Open University Press.

Martin, J. and Roberts, C. (1984) *Women and Employment: A Lifetime Perspective*, London: HMSO.

Millar, J. (1989) *Poverty and the Lone Parent: The Challenge to Social Policy*, Aldershot: Avebury.

—— (1994a) 'Lone parents and social security policy in the UK', in S. Baldwin and J. Falkingham (eds.) *Social Security and Social Change: New Challenges to the Beveridge Model*, Hemel Hempstead: Harvester Wheatsheaf.

—— (1994b) 'Family, state and personal responsibility: the changing balance for lone mothers in the UK', *Feminist Review* 48: 24–39.

—— (1996) 'Poor mothers and absent fathers', in H. Jones and J. Millar (eds.) *The Politics of the Family*, Aldershot: Avebury.

Millar, J. and Glendinning, C. (1989) 'Gender and poverty', *Journal of Social Policy* 18 (3): 363–82.

Millar, J. and Whiteford, P. (1993) 'Child support in lone-parent families: policies in Australia and the UK', *Policy and Politics* 21 (1): 59–72.

Millar, J., Leeper, S. and Davies, C. (1992) *Lone Parents, Poverty and Public Policy in Ireland,* Dublin: Combat Poverty Agency.

Mitchell, D. (1992) 'Sole parents, work and welfare: evidence from the Luxembourg Income Study', in S. Shaver (ed.) *Comparative Perspectives on Sole Parent Policy: Work and Welfare*, Proceedings of a seminar, University of New South Wales, Social Policy Research Centre.

Mitchell, J. (1975) *Psychoanalysis and Feminism*, Harmondsworth: Penguin.

Molyneux, M. (1985) 'Family reforms in socialist states: the hidden agenda', *Feminist Review* 21: 47–64.

Momsen, J.H. (1991) *Women and Development in the Third World* London and New York: Routledge.

Moore, H.L. (1994a) 'Social identities and the politics of reproduction', in *A Passion for Difference*, Cambridge: Polity Press.

—— (1994b) *Is There a Crisis in the Family?*, Geneva: United Nations Research Institute for Social Development.

Moore, H.L. and Vaughan, M. (1994) *Cutting Down Trees: Gender, Nutrition and Agricultural Change in the Northern Province of Zambia, 1890–1990*, Portsmouth, NJ: Heineman.

Morgan, P. (1995) *Farewell to the Family? Public Policy and the Family Breakdown in Britain and the USA*, London: Institute of Economic Affairs.

Morris, J. (ed.) (1992) *Alone Together: Voices of Single Mothers*, London: Women's Press.

Morris, L. (1990) *The Workings of the Household: A US–UK Comparison*, Cambridge: Polity Press.

—— (1994) *Dangerous Classes: The Underclass and Social Citizenship*, London: Routledge.

Moser, C (1994) 'Poverty and vulnerability in Chawama, Lusaka, Zambia 1978–1992', *Draft Research Paper*, Research Project on Urban Poverty and Social Policy in the Context of Adjustment, World Bank.

Moss, P. (1991) *Childcare in the European Community 1985–1990*, Brussels: EC Commission.

Muncie, J., Wetherell, M., Dallos, R. and Cochrane, A. (eds) (1995) *Understanding the Family*, London: Sage.

Murray, C. (1990) *The Emerging British Underclass*, London: Institute of Economic Affairs, Health and Welfare Unit.

—— (1993) 'The time has come to put a stigma back on illegitimacy', *Wall Street Journal*, 14 November.

Mwila, C. (1981) *Village People and Their Resources: An Observation of Some of the Major Socio-economic Characteristics of Rural Households in Mubanga, Chinsali District*, Lusaka: RDSB.

Myrdal, A. and Klein, V. (1956) *Women's Two Roles: Home and Work*, London: Routledge & Kegan Paul.

National Audit Office (1990) *Department of Social Security: Support for Lone Parent Families* (DSS/HoC 328), London: HMSO.

National Council for One Parent Families (1995) *Annual Report 1993–94. A Watershed Year for Lone Parents*, London: NCOPF.

Ní Bhrolcháin, M. (1992) 'Long-term effects of divorce: fact or fallacy?', *ESRC Data Archive Bulletin*, Colchester: University of Essex.

—— (1993) 'Outcomes Associated with Parental Divorce and Death: Further Discussion', *ESRC Data Archive Bulletin*, Colchester: University of Essex.

——(1994) 'Educational and socio-demographic outcomes among the children of disrupted and intact marriages', Department of Social Statistics, University of Southampton.

Niehaus, I. (1994) 'Disharmonious spouses and harmonious siblings: conceptualising household formation among urban residents in Qwaqwa', *African Studies* 53 (1).

Norton, C. (1982) *Caroline Norton's Defence*, Chicago: Academy; originally published 1854.

Nugent, J (1985) 'The old-age security motive for fertility', *Population and Development Review* 11 (1): 75–97.

OECD (1990) *Lone Parents: The Economic Challenge,* Paris: Organisation for Economic Co-operation and Development.

—— (1993) *Breadwinners or Child Rearers: The Dilemma for Lone Mothers*, Paris: Organisation for Economic Co-operation and Development.

Office of Population Censuses and Surveys (1994) *Marriage and Divorce Statistics 1992*, Series FM2, No. 20, London: HMSO.

Oldfield, N. and Yu, A.C.S. (1993) *The Cost of a Child*, London: Child Poverty Action Group.

Olwig, K.F. (1993), 'The migration experience: Nevisian women at home and abroad', in J.H. Momsen, (ed.) *Women and Change in the Caribbean*, Kingston, Jamaica: Ian Randle; London: James Currey.

Owen, D. (1994) *Ethnic Minority Women and the Labour Market: Analysis of the 1991 Census*, Manchester: Equal Opportunities Commission.

Parsons, T. and Bales, R. (1956) *Family Socialization and Interaction Process*, London: Routledge.

Perry, R. (1991) 'Colonizing the Breast: Sexuality and Maternity in Eighteenth Century England', *Journal of the History of Sexuality* 2 (2): 204–34.

Phipps-Yonas, S. (1980) 'Teenage pregnancy and motherhood: a review of the literature', *American Journal of Orthopsychiatry* 50 (3): 403–31.

Phizacklea, A. (1982) 'Migrant women and wage labour: the lives of West Indian women in Britain', in J. West (ed.) *Work, Women and the Labour Market*, London: Routledge & Kegan Paul.

Phoenix, A. (1987) 'Theories of gender and black families', in G. Weiner and

M. Arnot (eds) *Gender under Scrutiny: New Inquiries in Education*, London: Hutchinson.

—— (1988) 'Narrow definitions of culture: the case of early motherhood', in S. Westwood and P. Bhachu (eds) *Enterprising Women*, London: Routledge.

—— (1990) 'Black women and the maternity services', in J. Garcia, R. Kilpatrick and M. Richards (eds) *The Politics of Maternity Care*, Oxford: Clarendon.

—— (1991) *Young Mothers?*, Cambridge: Polity Press.

—— (1993) 'The social construction of teenage motherhood: a black and white issue?', in A. Lawson and D. Rhode (eds) *The Politics of Pregnancy: Adolescent Sexuality and Public Policy*, New Haven, Conn.: Yale University Press.

Pickup, L. (1988) 'Hard to get around: a study of women's travel mobility', in J. Little, L. Peake and P. Richardson (eds) *Women in Cities*, London: Macmillan.

Pinchbeck, I. (1930) *Women Workers and the Industrial Revolution, 1750–1850* (reprinted 1981, London: Virago).

Pithouse, A., Drury, C., and Butler, I. (1991) *Saint Mellons Child and Family Needs Survey: A Study Commissioned by South Glamorgan Social Services Department – Children and Families Services Section*, Cardiff: School of Social and Administrative Studies, University of Wales College of Cardiff.

Pollock, L. (1983) *Forgotten Children: Parent–Child Relations from 1500 to 1800*, Cambridge: Cambridge University Press.

Popay, J. and Jones, G. (1990) 'Patterns of health and illness amongst lone parents', *Journal of Social Policy* 19 (4): 499–534.

Population Reference Bureau (1992) *Chartbook: Africa Demographic and Health Surveys*, Washington, DC: Population Reference Bureau.

Preston-Whyte, E. (1993) 'Women who are not married: fertility, 'illegitimacy', and the nature of households and domestic groups among single African women in Durban', *South African Journal of Sociology* 24 (3): 63–71.

Pulsipher, L.M. (1993), 'Changing roles in the life cycles of women in traditional West Indian houseyards', in J.H. Momsen (ed.) *Women and Change in the Caribbean*, Kingston, Jamaica: Ian Randle; London: James Currey.

Prosser, W.R. (1991) 'The underclass: assessing what we have learned', *Focus* 13 (2): 1–18, Institute for Research on Poverty, University of Wisconsin-Madison.

Radford, J. (1991) 'Immaculate Conceptions', *Trouble and Strife* 21: 8–12.

Raffaelli, M. *et al.* (1991) 'Sexual practices and attitudes of street youth in Belo Horizonte, Brazil', *Social Science and Medicine* 37 (5): 661–70.

Rathbone, E. (1940) *The Case for Family Allowances*, Harmondsworth: Penguin.

Renvoize, J. (1985) *Going Solo: Single Mothers by Choice*, London: Routledge & Kegan Paul.

Ribbens, J. and Edwards, R. (1995) 'Introducing qualitative research on women in families and households', *Women's Studies International Forum*, Special Issue, 18: 3.

Richards, M. (1993) 'Why does parental divorce influence the lives of young adults?', presentation to the Marriage and Divorce seminar group, Bath University, June.

—— (1994) 'The Interests of Children at Divorce', paper presented at an international conference (Brussels) on 'Families and Justice', Edition Bruylant and the Librarie Générale de Droit et de Jurisprudence (1995, forthcoming) Paris.

Richards, M. and Elliott, B.J. (n.d.), Centre for Family Research, University of Cambridge, unpublished research reported in Burghes, L. (1994) *Lone Parenthood and Family Disruption: The Outcomes for Children*, London: Family Policy Studies Centre.

Riley, D. (1983) *War in the Nursery. Theories of the Child and Mother*, London: Virago.

Roberts, E. (1985) *A Woman's Place: An Oral History of Working-Class Women 1890–1940*, Oxford: Basil Blackwell.

Robinson, M. and Smith, D. (1993) *Step by Step: Focus on Stepfamilies*, London: Harvester Wheatsheaf.

Roll, J. (1992) *Lone-Parent Families in the European Community*, London: European Family and Social Policy Unit.

Roseneil, S. (1995) 'The coming of age of feminist sociology: some issues of practice and theory for the next twenty years', *British Journal of Sociology* 46 (2), June: 191–205.

Ross, E. (1986) 'Labour and love: rediscovering London's working-class mothers, 1870–1918', in J. Lewis (ed.) *Labour and Love: Women's Experience of Home and Family, 1850–1940*, Oxford: Basil Blackwell.

—— (1993) *Love and Toil: Motherhood in Outcast London, 1870–1918*, Oxford: Oxford University Press.

Rothman, B. (1994) 'Beyond mothers and fathers: ideology in a patriarchal society', in E.N. Glenn, G. Chang and L.R. Forcey (eds) *Mothering*, London: Routledge.

Rover, C. (1970) *Love, Morals and the Feminists*, London: Routledge & Kegan Paul.

Rowbotham, S. (1994) 'Strategies against sweated work in Britain, 1820–1920', in S. Rowbotham and S. Mitter (eds) *Dignity and Daily Bread: New Forms of Economic Organising Among Poor Women in the Third World and in the First*, London: Routledge.

Ruddick, S. (1980) 'Maternal thinking', *Feminist Studies* 6 (2): 342–67.

Sackmann, R. and Haüssermann, H. (1994) 'Do regions matter? Regional differences in female labour market participation in Germany', *The Diverse Worlds of European Patriarchy: Environment and Planning* 26 A(9): 1377–96.

Sainsbury, D. (1994) *Gendering Welfare States,* London: Sage.

Sauer, R. (1978) 'Infanticide and abortion in nineteenth-century Britain', *Population Studies* 32 (1): 81–93.

Schlachter, A.C. (1993) *India: The Forgotten Children of the Cities*, Florence: Innocenti Report, Unicef.

Scott-Jones, D. and Nelson-Le Gall, S. (1986) 'Defining black families: past and present', in E. Seidman and J. Rappaport (eds) *Redefining Social Problems*, New York: Plenum.

Scott, H. (1982) *Sweden's 'Right to be Human'*, London: Allison & Busby.

Seidman, E. and Rappaport, J. (1986) 'Framing the issues', in E. Seidman and J. Rappaport (eds) *Redefining Social Problems*, New York: Plenum.

Sen, A.K. (1981) *Poverty and Famines: An Essay on Entitlement and Deprivation* Oxford: Clarendon Press.

—— (1983) 'Economics and the family', *Asian Development Review* 1 (2): 14–26.

Sharpe, J. (1994) 'A world turned upside down: households and differentiation in a South African Bantustan in the 1990's, *African Studies* 53(1).

Sinclair, S.P. (1994) *Public Hostility Towards Lone Mothers*, paper presented at the Social Policy Association Annual Conference: 'Families in Question', University of Liverpool.

Slipman, S (1993) 'Who's left holding the baby?', *The Independent*, 6 July.

Smart, C. (1989) 'Power and the politics of child custody', in C. Smart and S. Sevenhuijsen (eds) *Child Custody and the Politics of Gender*, London: Routledge.

—— (ed.) (1992) *Regulating Womanhood*, London: Routledge.

—— (1996) 'Good wives and moral lives: marriage and divorce 1937–51', in C. Gledhill and G. Swanson (eds) *Nationalising Femininity*, Manchester: Manchester University Press.

Smart, C. and Brophy, J. (1985) 'Locating law: a discussion of the place of law in feminist politics', in J. Brophy J and C. Smart (eds) *Women in Law*, London: Routledge.

Smart, C. and Sevenhuijsen, S. (eds) (1989) *Child Custody and the Politics of Gender*, London: Routledge.

*Social Trends* (various years, 1980s and 1990s), London: Central Statistical Office.

Solinger, R. (1994) 'Race and value: black and white illegitimate babies, 1945–65', in E. N. Glenn, G. Chang and L. R. Forcey (eds) *Mothering: Ideology, Experience and Agency*, New York: Routledge.

Somerville, J. (1992) 'The New Right and family politics', *Economy and Society* 21 (2): 93–128.

Sontag, S. (1983) *Illness as Metaphor*, Harmondsworth: Penguin.

Spensky, M. (1989) 'From the Workhouse to the home for unmarried mothers: a feminist perspective', paper presented at the British Sociological Association Annual Conference, Plymouth Polytechnic.

—— (1992) 'Producers of legitimacy: homes for unmarried mothers in the 1950s', in C. Smart (ed.) *Regulating Womanhood*, London: Routledge.

Stacey, J. (1983) *Patriarchy and Socialist Revolution in China*, Berkeley: University of California Press.

—— (1994) 'Scents, scholars and stigma: the revisionist campaign for family values', *Social Text* 40: 51–75.

Stanworth, M. (1987) 'Reproductive technologies and the deconstruction of motherhood', in M. Stanworth (ed.) *Reproductive Technologies: Gender, Motherhood and Medicine*, Cambridge: Polity Press.

*Statistical Report of the Nordic Countries* (1987), Copenhagen: Nordic Statistical Secretariat.

Stivens, M. (1987) 'Family and state in Malaysian industrialisation: the case of Rembau, Negeri Sembilan, Malaysia', in H. Afshar (ed.) *Women, State and Ideology,* London: Macmillan.

Summerfield, P. (1984) *Women Workers in the Second World War: Production and Patriarchy in Conflict,* London: Routledge.

Swann, Lord (1985) *Education for All: Committee of Inquiry into the Education of Children from Ethnic Minority Groups,* London: HMSO.

Swift, A (1993) *Brazil: The Fight for Childhood in the City,* Florence: Innocenti Report, Unicef.

Szanton Blanc (1994) *Urban Children in Distress: Global Predicaments and Strategies,* New York: Gordon & Breach.

ten Tusscher, T. (1986) 'Patriarchy, capitalism and the New Right', in J. Evans *et al.* (eds) *Feminism and Political Theory,* London: Sage.

Thane, P. (1978) 'Women and the Poor Law in Victorian and Edwardian England', *History Workshop Journal* 6: 20–51.

Thomas, D. (1990) 'Intra-household resource allocation: an inferential approach', *Journal of Human Resources* 25 (4): 635–64.

Thornton Dill, B. (1988) 'Our mother's grief: racial ethnic women and the maintenance of families', *Journal of Family History* 13: 415–31.

*Times, The* (1991) 'One-parent homes blamed for school problems', 2 August.

Titmus, R. (1976) *Essays on the Welfare State,* London: Allen & Unwin (1st edn 1958).

Tracey, L. (1994) 'Motherhood and social policy in York, 1950–1955', MA dissertation, University of Warwick.

Trebilcot, J. (1983) *Mothering: Essays in Feminist Theory,* Savage, Md.: Rowman & Littlefield.

UNDP (1994) *Human Development Report 1994,* Oxford: Oxford University Press.

United Nations (1989) *1987 Demographic Yearbook,* New York: United Nations Publications.

—— (1992) *1991 Demographic Yearbook,* New York: United Nations Publications.

—— (1993) *Demographic Yearbook: Special Issue on Population, Ageing and the Situation of Elderly Persons,* New York: United Nations Publications.

—— (1994) *1992 Demographic Yearbook,* New York: United Nations Publications.

Utting, D., Bright, J. and Henricson, C. (1993) *Crime and the Family: Improving Child-rearing and Preventing Delinquency,* Occasional paper 16, London: Family Policy Studies Centre.

Van Driel, F. (1994) *Poor and Powerful: Female-Headed Households and Unmarried Mothers in Botswana,* Nijmegen: NICCOS.

Vickery, A. (1993) 'Golden Age to separate spheres? A review of the categories and chronology of English women's history', Historiographical Review, *The Historical Journal* 36 (2): 383–414.

Wahrman, D. (1993) 'Middle-class domesticity goes public: gender, class, and politics from Queen Caroline to Queen Victoria', *Journal of British Studies* 32: 396–432.

Walby, S. (1986) *Patriarchy at Work: Patriarchy and Capitalist Relations in Employment,* Cambridge: Polity Press.

—— (1990) *Theorizing Patriarchy,* Oxford: Blackwell.

—— (1993) ' "Backlash" in historical context', in M. Kennedy, C. Lubelska and V. Walsh (eds) *Making Connections: Women's Studies, Women's Movements, Women's Lives*, London: Taylor & Francis.

Walker, I. (1990) 'The effects of income support measures on the labour market behaviour of lone mothers', *Fiscal Studies* 11: 55–78.

Wallerstein, J. and Blakeslee, S. (1989) *Second Chances*, London, Bantam Press.

Ward, M. (1986) *Poor Women, Powerful Men: America's Great Experiment in Family Planning*, Boulder, Colo.: Westview Press.

Weitzman, L. (1985) *The Divorce Revolution: The Unexpected Social and Economic Consequences for Women and Children in America*, New York: Free Press.

Wennemo, I. (1994) *Sharing the Costs of Children: Studies on the Development of Family Support in OECD Countries*, Stockholm: Swedish Institute for Social Research Dissertation Series.

Whatmore, S. (1991) *Farming Women: Gender, Work and Family Enterprises*, London: Macmillan.

Whiteford, P. and Bradshaw, J. (1994) 'Benefits and incentives for lone parents: a comparative analysis', *International Social Security Review* 47 (3/4): 69–90.

Wilensky, H.L. (1975) *The Welfare State and Equality: Structural and Ideological Roots of Public Expenditure*, Berkeley: University of California Press.

Willard Williams, C. (1990) *Black Teenage Mothers: Pregnancy and Childrearing from their Perspective*, Lexington, Mass.: Lexington Books.

Williams, F. (1989) *Social Policy: A Critical Introduction, Issues of Race, Gender and Class*, Cambridge, Polity Press.

Willmott, P. and Young, M. (1960) *Family and Class in a London Suburb*, London: Routledge & Kegan Paul.

Wilson, W.J. (1987) *The Truly Disadvantaged: The Inner City, the Underclass and Public Policy*, Chicago: University of Chicago Press.

Wilson, J.Q. (1993) *The Moral Sense*, New York: Free Press.

Wimbush, E. and Talbot, M. (eds) (1988) *Relative Freedoms: Women and Leisure*, Milton Keynes: Open University Press.

Winnicott, D. (1953) 'Review of Bowlby's *Maternal Care and Mental Health*', in C. Winnicott, R. Shepherd and M. Davis (eds) (1989) *D.W. Winnicott: Psycho-Analytic Explorations*, Cambridge, Mass.: Harvard University Press.

—— (1957) *The Child, the Family, and the Outside World*, reprinted 1971, Harmondsworth: Penguin.

—— (1960) 'Ego distortion in terms of true and false self', in D.W. Winnicott (1965) *The Maturational Processes and the Facilitating Environment. Studies in the Theory of Emotional Development*, London: Hogarth Press.

—— (1967) 'The concept of clinical regression compared with that of defence organisation', in C. Winnicott, R. Shepherd and M. Davis (eds) (1989) *D.W. Winnicott: Psycho-Analytic Explorations*, Cambridge, Mass.: Harvard University Press.

Wong, Y., Garfinkel, I. and McLanahan, S. (1992) *Single-Mother Families in*

*Eight Countries: Economic Status and Social Policy*, University of Wisconsin–Madison: Institute for Research on Poverty.

World Bank (1993) *World Development Report 1993: Investing in Health*, Washington, DC: World Bank.

Wright, C. (1993) 'Unemployment, migration and changing gender relations in Lesotho', PhD dissertation, University of Leeds.

Wylie, I. (1995) 'Hard cases alter bad law', *Guardian*, 28 January.

Yeboah, Y. (1991) 'Equal opportunities for women: the implications of adolescent pregnancy and childbirth in sub-saharan Africa for ILO policies and programmes', Geneva: International Labour Organisation.

Young, I. (1983) 'Is male gender identity the cause of male domination?', in J. Trebilcot (ed.) *Mothering*, Savage, Md.: Rowman & Littlefield.

Younge, G. (1995) 'Black in Britain', *Guardian*, 20 March.

Youssef, N. and Hetler, C. (1983) 'Establishing the economic conditions of women-headed households in the Third World: a new approach', in M. Buvinic and M. Lycette (eds) *Women's Issues in Third World Poverty*, Baltimore: Johns Hopkins University Press.

Ziegler, D. (1995) 'Single parenting: a visual analysis', in B. Dickerson (ed.) *African American Single Mothers: Understanding their Lives and Families*, London: Sage.

# Index